INTERPRETING CARDIAC ARRHYTHMIAS

Mary Brambilla McFarland, B.S.N., M.S.N.
Assistant Professor, Department of Nursing
Columbus College, Columbus, Georgia

© Springer Publishing Company, Inc. 1975

All rights reserved. No part of this publication may be reproduced or transmitted, in any form or by any means, without prior permission

First published in the U.S.A. in 1975 by
Springer Publishing Company, Inc.
200 Park Avenue South, New York, NY 10003

First published in the U.K. in 1978 by
THE MACMILLAN PRESS LTD
London and Basingstoke
Associated companies in Delhi Dublin
Hong Kong Johannesburg Lagos Melbourne
New York Singapore and Tokyo

Printed in Hong Kong

British Library Cataloguing in Publication Data

McFarland, Mary Brambilla
    Interpreting cardiac arrhythmias

    1. Arrhythmia – Diagnosis   2. Electrocardiography
    3. Cardiovascular disease nursing
    I. Title
    616.1'28'0754   RC674

ISBN 0-333-25514-3

The paperback edition of this book is sold subject to the condition that it shall not, by way of trade or otherwise, be lent, resold, hired out, or otherwise circulated without the publisher's prior consent in any form of binding or cover other than that in which it is published and without a similar condition including this condition being imposed on the subsequent purchaser

This book is sold subject to the standard conditions of the Net Book Agreement

To the memory of my father,
Mario Brambilla

CONTENTS

Foreword   vii

1. **Anatomy and Physiology of the Heart   1**
   Location   1
   Structure   3
       Chambers and valves   4 / Coronary circulation   6
   The Conduction System   9
   Electrophysiology (Action Potential)   11
       Depolarization   11 / Repolarization   12 / Relationship of the action potential to the cardiac cycle   13

2. **The Electrocardiogram   15**
   The Leads of the Electrocardiogram   16
       Bipolar standard leads   16 / Unipolar augmented extremity leads   17 / Unipolar chest leads   18
   The ECG Paper   19
   The ECG Pattern   19
       The P wave   20 / The P-R interval   20 / The QRS complex   21 / The S-T segment   21 / The T wave   21 / The U wave   22

v

3. **Arrhythmias** 23

   Interpretation of ECG Patterns 23
   Classification of Arrhythmias 25
   Identification of Arrhythmias 27
   Sinus arrhythmias 28 / *Atrial arrhythmias* 33 / *Junctional (nodal) arrhythmias* 44 / *Ventricular arrhythmias* 50
   Conduction Defects 58
   First degree heart block 58 / *Second degree heart block* 60 / *Complete heart block (third degree)* 62
   Some Sample Rhythm Strips 64

4. **Pacemakers** 71

   Definition and Historical Development 71
   Uses 72
   Types of Pacemaker Units (Pulse Generators) 72
   External 72 / *Internal* 74
   Pacemaker Rates 74
   Pacemaker Electrodes 76
   Epicardial electrodes 76 / *Endocardial electrodes* 78 / *Transthoracic electrodes* 80
   Nursing Care of Patients with Pacemakers 81

Self Test 91
Selected Readings 112
Glossary 115

FOREWORD

Ten years ago most nurses could neither understand nor interpret electrocardiograph tracings. Today, curricula for all nursing education programs include instruction in this aspect of patient care. The purpose of this book is to help meet the need for a simplified approach to the electrocardiographic interpretation of arrhythmias. While it is intended primarily for use by students in undergraduate nursing programs, it may also be useful to the practitioner who wishes to review the fundamentals of the electrocardiographic representation of cardiac arrhythmias.

Mary Brambilla McFarland

CHAPTER 1

Anatomy and Physiology of the Heart

LOCATION

The heart does not lie in the anatomical position in which it is usually described. The *right side* of the heart is actually in an anterior position and is protected by the sternum. It is almost directly in front of the portion of the heart described as the *left side,* which lies in a posterior position close to the vertebral column. The heart is approximately the size of the same individual's closed fist. The broad top, or base, points upward, posteriorly, and to the right; the narrow bottom, or apex, points downward, anteriorly, and to the left. As a result, the anatomical axis runs from the apex upward and backward at an

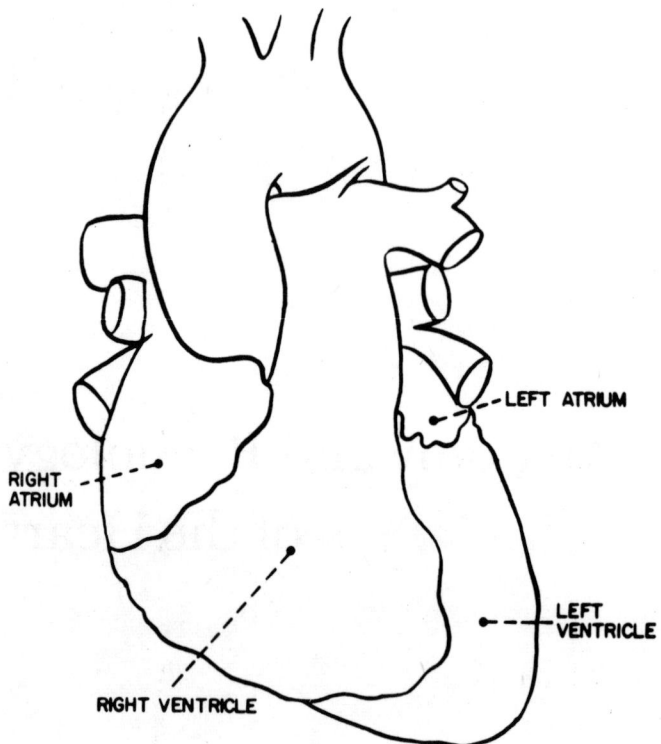

Figure 1-1. Anatomical position of the heart.

angle of about 30° from the horizontal plane (Figure 1-2). The heart is not attached to surrounding organs but is kept in its proper position by the great blood vessels in the thorax and by the membranous sac that encloses it — the pericardium.

ANATOMY AND PHYSIOLOGY OF THE HEART

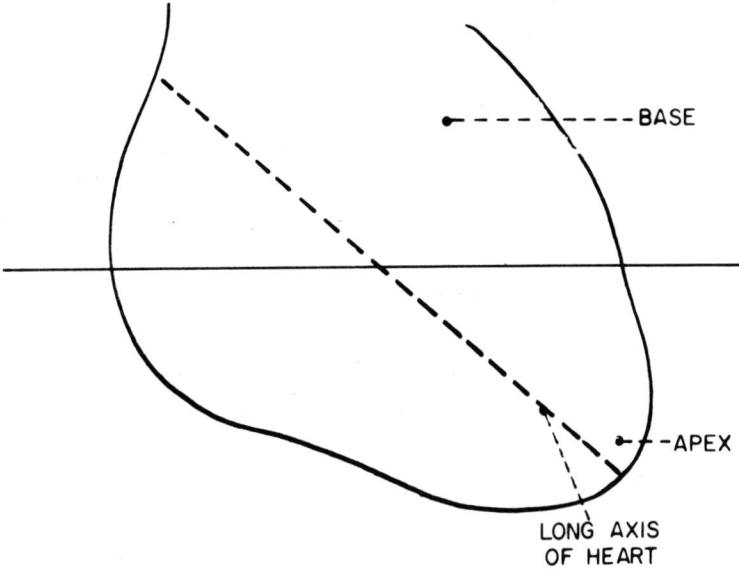

Figure 1-2. The long axis of the heart.

STRUCTURE

The heart is a hollow, muscular organ composed of three layers, the *pericardium* (outer layer), the *myocardium* (middle layer), and the *endocardium* (inner layer). The pericardium is a fibroserous sac that surrounds the heart. It is composed of two membranes, an external fibrous membrane and a serous membrane. On the upper surface of the heart the fibrous membrane extends onto the great vessels covering them for 1½ inches; on the lower surface it is attached to the diaphragm; and on the anterior surface it is attached to the sternum. The serous part of the membrane is a closed sac consisting of a parietal layer that lines the fibrous membrane and a visceral layer, called the epicardium, that covers the heart. Although these two membranes are in contact with each other, they are freely movable;

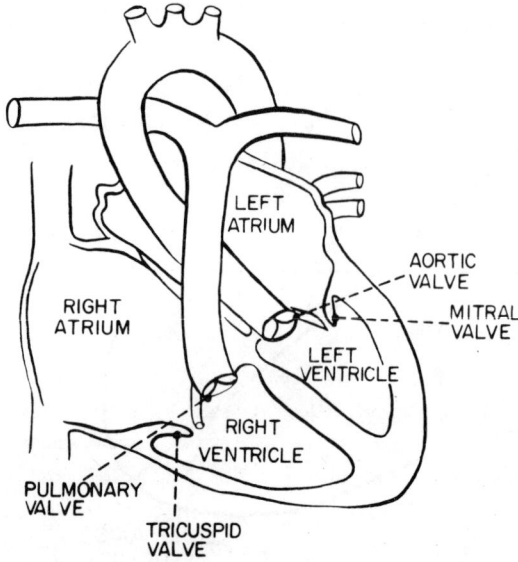

Figure 1-3. Chambers and valves of the heart.

the small amount of pericardial fluid that is present between them lubricates their surfaces and prevents friction from occurring when the heart muscle contracts.

The myocardium is composed of layers and bundles of specialized muscle tissue that form the walls of the atria and ventricles and also include the conduction system of the heart.

The endocardium is the smooth, thin, inner lining of the heart. It lines the atria and ventricles and covers the valves (see Figure 1-3).

Chambers and Valves

The heart consists of four chambers, an atrium and a ventricle located on the right (or anterior) side of the heart and an atrium and a ventricle located on the left (or posterior) side of the heart.

ANATOMY AND PHYSIOLOGY OF THE HEART

The right atrium receives unoxygenated, venous blood from three sources:
1. The superior vena cava delivers blood from the head and arms.
2. The inferior vena cava delivers blood from the abdomen and legs.
3. The coronary sinus drains venous blood from the myocardial blood vessels.

When the right atrium becomes filled with blood, the blood volume exerts pressure on the tricuspid valve, which then opens and allows the blood to flow into the right ventricle. The leaflets of this three-cusped valve are composed of strong fibrous tissue and their bases are attached to a fibrous ring that surrounds the opening between the right atrium and ventricle. The apices and margins of the cusps are anchored in the muscular wall of the ventricle by chordae tendinae, strong fibrous cords that are attached to the papillary muscles. The papillary muscles are conical muscular projections from the wall and septum of the heart.

When the right ventricle has filled, pressure is exerted on the under side of the three opened leaflets of the tricuspid valve causing it to close and prevent blood from flowing in the opposite direction, i.e., back into the atrium. The papillary muscles prevent the leaflets from inverting into the atrium when the ventricle contracts.

When the right ventricle, which has a muscle mass three times as thick as that of the right atrium, contracts, the semilunar valve that guards the opening into the pulmonary artery opens, and the venous blood is pumped into the pulmonary artery which carries it to the lungs through its right and left branches. The oxygenated blood then returns to the left atrium of the heart via four pulmonary veins.

The left atrium is distinctly thicker than the right atrium and has a somewhat irregular area on the otherwise smooth surface of the septum, indicating the position of the fetal foramen ovale (fossa ovalis). As the left atrium fills, pressure on the

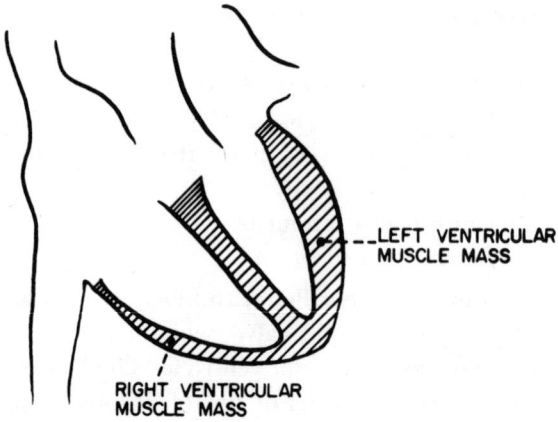

Figure 1-4. The ventricular muscle mass.

bicuspid (mitral) valve forces it to open and blood flows into the left ventricle. The bicuspid valve is similar to the tricuspid valve in structure and function, except that it has two rather than three cusps.

The average thickness of the left ventricle is three times that of the right ventricle — a muscle mass necessary to carry out its heavy workload. Its inner surface, like that of the right ventricle, gives rise to papillary muscles and chordae tendinae that are attached to the mitral valve cusps.

Finally, the oxygenated (arterial) blood is pumped by the left ventricle into the aorta, the opening of which is guarded by the three-cusped aortic valve, and thence into the general circulation.

Coronary Circulation

Oxygenated blood is carried to the myocardium by two main coronary arteries that arise at the cusps of the aortic valve and encircle the heart like a crown (corona) (Figures 1-5, 1-6).

ANATOMY AND PHYSIOLOGY OF THE HEART

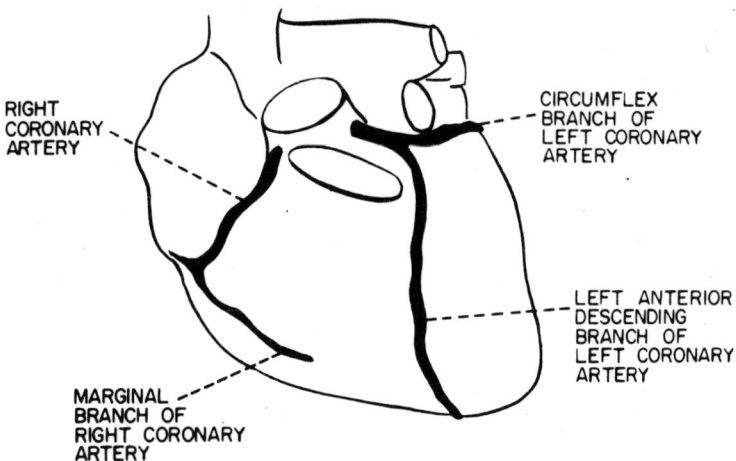

Figure 1-5. Anterior view — coronary circulation.

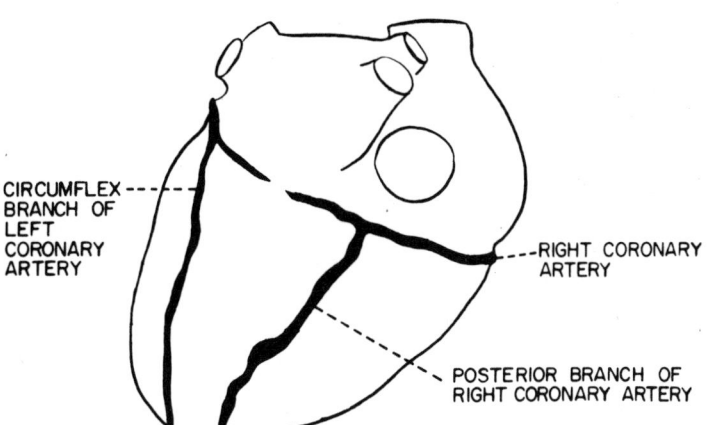

Figure 1-6. Posterior view — coronary circulation.

The right coronary artery, originating from the right aortic sinus, passes to the right side of the heart, under the right atrium to the sulcus (or groove) between the right atrium and the right ventricle. It divides into two branches, the marginal branch and the posterior descending branch. The marginal branch descends to the apex of the heart where it supplies both the anterior and posterior surfaces of the right ventricle. The posterior descending branch of the right coronary artery gives off a small branch to the atrioventricular node before it descends to the posterior sulcus where it supplies adjacent portions of both the right and left ventricles.

The left coronary artery, originating in the left aortic sinus, passes to the left side of the heart, under the left atrium and separates into two main divisions, the anterior descending branch and the circumflex branch. The anterior descending branch supplies the interventricular septum, the anterior surface of the left ventricle and the lateral margin of the left ventricle. The posterior surface of the left ventricle is supplied by the circumflex branch. The right and left coronary arteries have branches that anastomose (come together) on the posterior surface of the heart forming a crown.

The coronary veins return venous blood from the heart muscle to the right atrium. These veins encircle the heart parallel to the coronary arteries and terminate in the coronary sinus which opens into the right atrium between the tricuspid valve and the inferior vena cava.

THE CONDUCTION SYSTEM

The heart has a conduction system that originates its own electrical stimulus and transmits it through specialized muscle fibers. This system consists of: (1) the sinoatrial (S-A) node; (2) the internodal atrial pathways; and (3) the Purkinje system, which includes: (a) the atrioventricular junction (A-V node); (b) the atrioventricular bundle (bundle of His); (c) the right and left bundle branches; and (d) terminal fibers called Purkinje fibers.

The sinoatrial node is located in the wall of the right atrium near the entrance of the superior vena cava. It is an area of muscle cells that is able to initiate a heart beat 75-80 times per minute. The S-A node is called the pacemaker of the heart because, under normal conditions, no other area of the heart is able to generate impulses as rapidly as this node. In certain

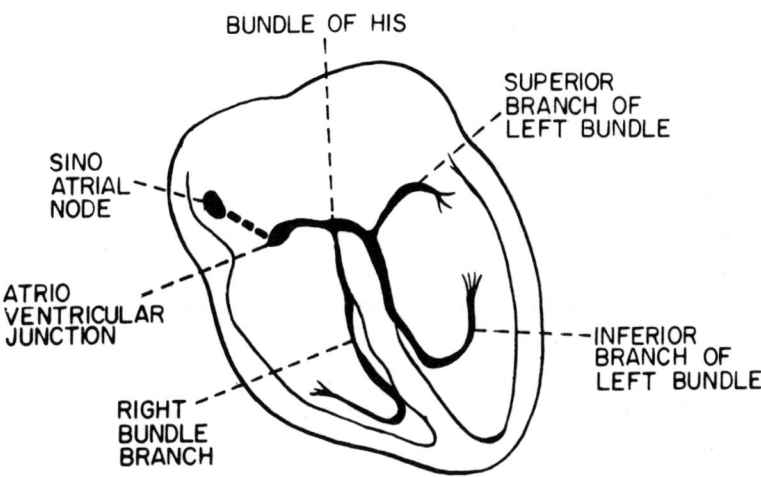

Figure 1-7.   The conduction system of the heart.

pathologic states, however, other portions of the heart muscle may take over this pacemaking function. For example, the A-V node can pace the heart at a rate of 40-50 beats per minute.

The electrical impulse that originates in the S-A node spreads through the muscles of the atria causing them to contract. Following atrial excitation, the wave of conduction spreads to the Purkinje system. The atrioventricular node, consisting of specialized neuromuscular tissue, is located on the right side of the interatrial septum near the entrance of the inferior vena cava. The A-V node slows the conduction wave as it passes from the atria to the ventricles. This delay provides time for complete contraction of the atria prior to stimulation of the ventricles. The impulse then passes from the A-V node to the bundle of His, which is located in the upper portion of the interventricular septum. The lower portion of the bundle of His divides into the right and left bundle branches. The right bundle branch, which carries the impulse to the right ventricle, is the longer of the two. The left bundle branch carries the impulse to the left ventricle where it divides into a superior and inferior branch. These bundle branches terminate in the Purkinje fibers that carry the impulse to the lateral walls of the ventricles causing them to contract.

After contracting, the cardiac muscle rests and recovers. The atrial recovery phase occurs during the contraction of the ventricles. Ventricular recovery takes place before the next stimulus is sent out by the S-A node. The combined periods of contraction and recovery constitute the cardiac cycle, which lasts about 0.8 second.

The automaticity and rhythmicity of this cycle depend upon the ability of the specialized cells of the conduction system to generate and transmit impulses. The initial pacemaking stimulus in the S-A node depends upon the presence in the blood of sodium, potassium, and calcium, and on energy such as that provided by the oxidation of glucose. The mechanism by which these specialized cells fire is the action potential.

ELECTROPHYSIOLOGY (ACTION POTENTIAL)

The distribution of ions along the inside and outside of a cell membrane affects the ability of that cell to transmit electrical impulses. The most important of these ions are sodium and potassium. Sodium ions (Na+) are in greatest number outside of the cell while potassium ions (K+) predominate within the cell. In addition, the number of positively charged sodium ions around the outside of the cell is *greater than* the number of positively charged potassium ions inside the cell. This means that the inside of the cell has less positive charges than the outside and, therefore, is considered to be negatively charged *relative* to the outside of the cell. A cell at this stage is polarized and in a state of resting potential.

Depolarization

When a resting cell is stimulated there is an abrupt increase in the size of the pores along the cell membrane. Once received, the stimulus flows across the surface of the cell in a wave-like manner increasing the permeability of the cell-wall membrane and thus allowing sodium ions to rush to the inside and potassium ions to rush out of the cell. As a result, the number of sodium ions is greater inside the cell and potassium ions are in greater concentration on the outside. The polarity of the cell membrane is reversed and the inside of the cell has become positive *relative* to the outside. When this has occurred, the cell is depolarized and muscular contraction results. This process of depolarization may be stated as:

    stimulation → depolarization → muscular contraction

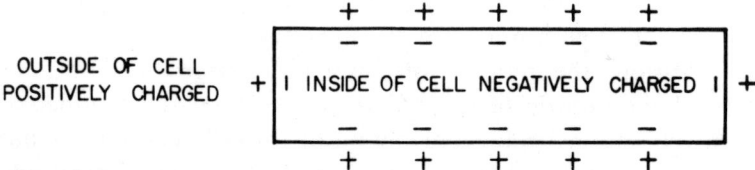

a.

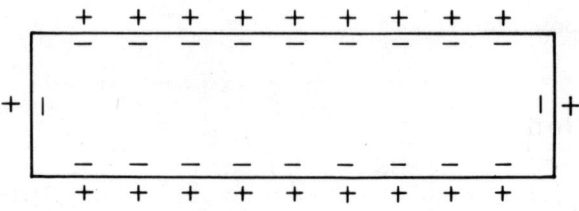

b.

c.

Figure 1-8. The electrophysiology of cells. a. Distribution of ions. b. Resulting electrical charge. c. Polarized cell in the

Repolarization

Following depolarization, the muscle cell reestablishes its resting potential. The mechanism by which this occurs is not clearly understood. However, it is known that a sodium pump stimulated by metabolic activity forces sodium ions back across the cell membrane. Potassium also moves to the inside and the polarity of the cell is reestablished.

ANATOMY AND PHYSIOLOGY OF THE HEART 13

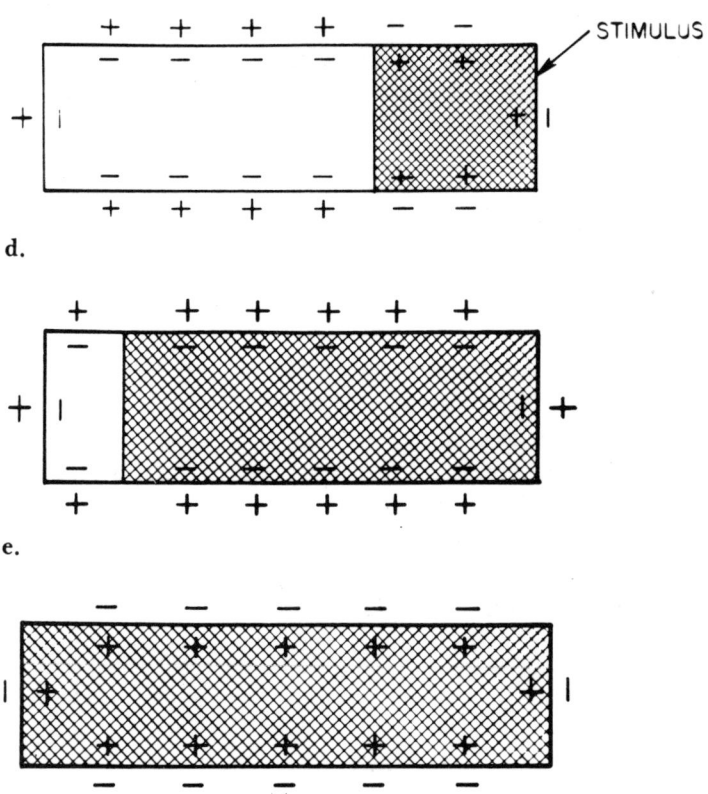

resting state. d. Cell upon stimulation. e. Flow of stimulus across cell membrane. f. Depolarized cell.

Relationship of the Action Potential to the Cardiac Cycle

The cells in the S-A node are inherently capable of self-excitation. The cell membrane of the S-A node slowly allows sodium ions to passively diffuse into the cell. As a result, the potential difference in ionic balance between the inside and outside of the cell changes. The pacemaker cell becomes more and more positive inside until a state of self-excitation is reached. At this point, a sudden increase in membrane permeability occurs; depolarization begins and subsequently travels throughout the conduction system. Following depolarization, the muscle cells of the heart must become repolarized and return to the resting state before they can accept another stimulus. If the cells are stimulated before complete repolarization has occurred they will not be able to accept the stimulus. As this point the cells are said to be in a refractory state.

Because the conduction of impulses through the heart occurs in a wave-like manner, there are periods of time when some of the cells are resting and able to accept a stimulus. These cells are said to be in a nonrefractory state. At the same time, other cells, which are becoming depolarized, are unable to accept another impulse, and are said to be in a refractory state. If the heart receives a very strong stimulus (such as a powerful electrical current) during this time, the normally rhythmic electrical conduction will become chaotic because the nonrefractory cells will be accepting the stimulus while the refractory cells are rejecting it.

CHAPTER 2

The Electrocardiogram

The electrocardiogram (ECG) is a graphic representation of the electrical activity of the heart. Many of the changes in electrical impulses that occur throughout the cardiac cycle can be recorded by applying electrodes to various positions on the surface of the body and connecting them to an electrocardiograph machine. Each of these electrodes records the activity of the heart from a different position. The standard placement of electrodes is as follows:
   1. On the right arm — to convey the electrical forces of the heart from the position of the right shoulder.
   2. On the left arm — to convey the electrical forces of the heart from the position of the left shoulder.

3. On the left leg—to convey the electrical forces on the diaphragmatic (or lower) surface of the heart as the impulses are transmitted through the body tissues to the left hip.
4. On the right leg—to function as a ground; this electrode has no role in recording the electrical forces of the heart.
5. An exploring electrode is placed in one of six different positions on the chest (V_1-V_6) to convey electrical forces of the heart from those various positions.

THE LEADS OF THE ELECTROCARDIOGRAM

A lead is composed of both a positive and negative electrode. A *bipolar* lead is recorded when both electrodes are located on the body's surface. A *unipolar* lead is recorded when the positive electrode is on the body surface alone and is not influenced by another electrode.

By turning the lead selector switch on the ECG machine, 12 lead positions can be recorded.

Bipolar Standard Leads

Einthoven's triangle illustrates the placement and relationship of the three bipolar standard limb leads:

Standard lead I   Records the difference of electrical potential between the left arm and the right arm.

Standard lead II Records the difference of electrical potential between the left leg (or foot) and the right arm.

THE ELECTROCARDIOGRAM

Standard lead III Records the difference of electrical potential between the left leg and the left arm.

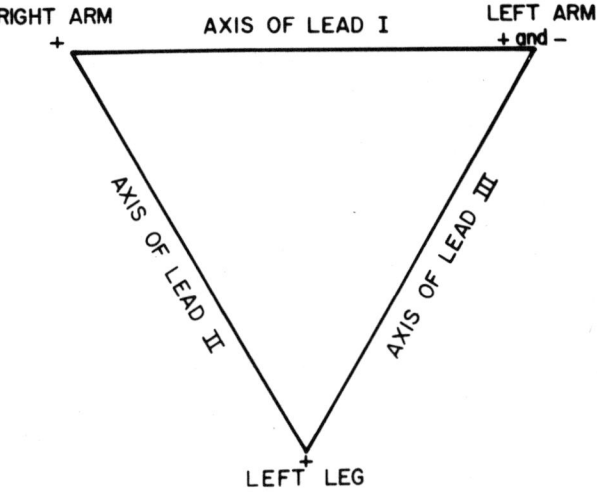

Figure 2-1. Einthoven's triangle.

Unipolar Augmented Extremity Leads

Three augmented unipolar leads are derived by eliminating the negative electrode. The resulting energy is known as *augmented voltage*. These three leads are:

    aVR (augmented voltage right)   The recording of right arm electrical forces.
    aVL (augmented voltage left)   The recording of left arm electrical forces.
    aVF (augmented voltage foot)   The recording of left leg (or foot) electrical forces.

Unipolar Chest Leads

The chest or V leads (V_1-V_6) record the electrical potentials at the following six chest positions:

- V_1 Fourth intercostal space at the right sternal border.
- V_2 Fourth intercostal space at the left sternal border.
- V_3 Midway between V_2 and V_4.
- V_4 Fifth intercostal space in the mid-clavicular line.
- V_5 Anterior axillary line on the same level as V_4.
- V_6 Mid-axillary line on the same level as V_4 and V_5.

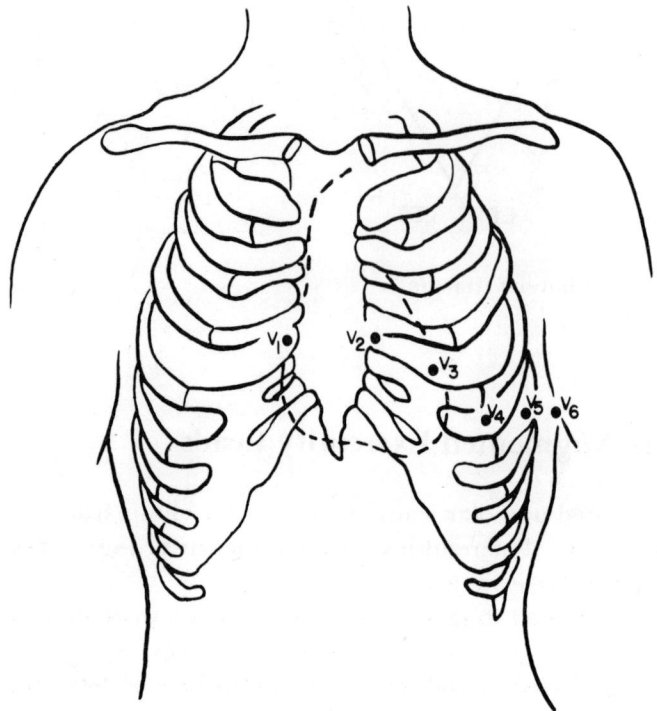

Figure 2-2. Locations for placement of electrodes for unipolar chest leads.

THE ECG PAPER

The ECG paper is marked with horizontal and vertical lines 1 mm apart. Every fifth line is heavier than the others, both horizontally and vertically, making squares that measure 5 mm in both directions.
   The vertical lines measure voltage:
      One small square (1 mm) equals 0.1 millivolt.
   The horizontal lines measure time:
      One small square (1 mm) equals 0.04 seconds.
      One large square (5 mm) equals 0.2 seconds.
   The short vertical lines in the upper margin of the ECG paper are placed at 3-second (75 mm) intervals and are used to quickly estimate the heart rate. The number of ventricular complexes in a 3-second strip multiplied by 20 gives the approximate rate for 1 minute. This rate may also be calculated by counting the number of ventricular complexes on a 6-second strip and multiplying that number by 10.

THE ECG PATTERN

The following description of the normal ECG pattern will be in reference to the ECG standard lead II. This lead was chosen because it is the most versatile for identifying arrhythmias and is the lead most commonly used for cardiac monitoring.
   The electrical activity of the heart that is recorded by the ECG is characterized by six wave deflections, designated by the letters P, Q, R, S, T, and U, each representing one phase of the cardiac cycle (see Figure 2-3).

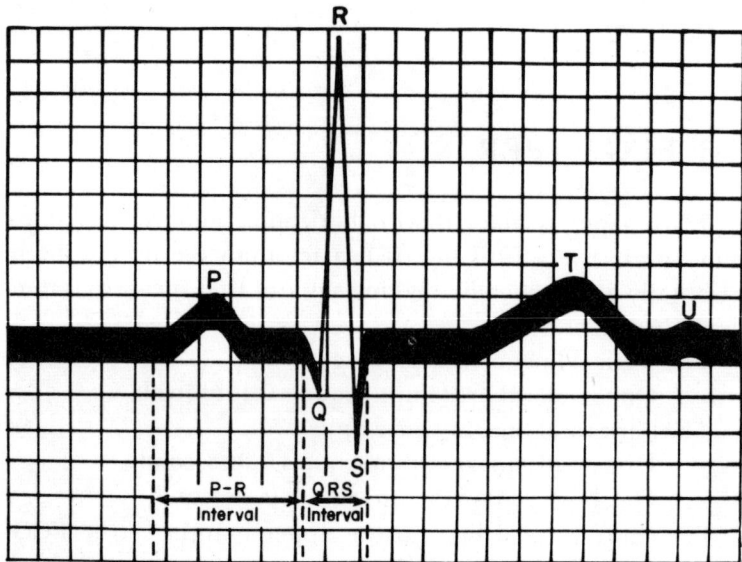

Figure 2-3. Normal P wave and QRS interval.

The P Wave

The P wave represents the electrical conduction through the atria. It is produced by the impulse that originates in the S-A node and subsequently spreads throughout both atria, the right atrium being activated approximately 0.01 seconds before the left. The P wave is a wave of atrial depolarization and is the first positive deflection seen on the ECG.

The P-R Interval

The P-R interval represents the time it takes for the original impulse to traverse the atria and delay in the A-V node. It is measured from the start of the P wave (atrial depolarization) to the beginning of the QRS complex (ventricular depolarization).

In an adult, the normal P-R interval ranges between 0.12 seconds to 0.20 seconds. There may be a slight variation of this value depending on the heart rate. At a heart rate less than 60, the P-R interval may be prolonged to 0.22 seconds and be normal, whereas a P-R interval of 0.20 with a heart rate above 100 may be of clinical significance.

The QRS Complex

The QRS complex represents depolarization of the ventricles. The Q wave correlates with the initial downward or negative deflection following the P wave and represents the beginning of ventricular depolarization. The R wave represents the first upward or positive deflection during ventricular depolarization. The S wave represents the first negative deflection following the R wave and completes the QRS complex and ventricular depolarization. The normal duration of the QRS complex (measured from the beginning of the Q wave to the end of the S wave) should not normally exceed 0.10 seconds.

The S-T Segment

The time interval represented by the S-T segment correlates with the resting period between ventricular depolarization and repolarization. During this time interval, which is also called the refractory period, the heart muscle cannot respond to stimuli.

The T Wave

The T wave represents the recovery phase after contraction (ventricular repolarization). Although it normally correlates with a positive deflection, changes in its shape occur frequently and are not necessarily indicative of heart disease.

The U Wave

The U wave represents a positive deflection following the T wave and is very difficult to identify on the standard lead II of the ECG. The exact cause of this wave is not known. Some believe that it represents the result of slow repolarization of the intraventricular conduction system.

CHAPTER 3

Arrhythmias

INTERPRETATION OF ECG PATTERNS

The initial preliminary recognition of cardiac arrhythmias is often made by the nurse who is watching a cardiac monitor. However, accurate confirmation and documentation of arrhythmias is made by evaluating and interpreting the abnormality on an electrocardiographic recording of the patient's heartbeats. The evaluation of this recording, often referred to as a "rhythm strip," must be done systematically. The following five steps will help the nurse to properly interpret and identify abnormalities in the cardiac rate, rhythm, and/or conduction.

1. Calculate the ventricular heart rate. This may be done in one of the following ways.
    a. Count the number of QRS complexes in a 6-inch strip and multiply by 10.
    b. Count the number of large squares between two R waves and divide that number into 300. (This method can only be used if the rhythm is regular.)

For example:
- 1 large square = rate of 300
- 2 large squares = rate of 150
- 3 large squares = rate of 100
- 4 large squares = rate of 75
- 5 large squares = rate of 60

   c. For a very fast rhythm, count the number of small squares between R waves and divide that number into 1500. (This method too can only be used when the rhythm is regular.)

2. Determine the rhythm of the R waves by measuring and comparing the time interval between these waves. If the R waves occur regularly with a variance of less than 0.12 seconds (3 small squares) between waves the ventricular rhythm is normal. A greater variance indicates an irregular ventricular rhythm, which may be slighly irregular, regularly irregular, or grossly irregular.

   Slightly irregular rhythms are characterized by only a minimal variance in the R-R intervals.

   Regularly irregular rhythms occur when the irregularity is systematic and predictable, though an irregular rhythm has been established.

   Grossly irregular rhythms occur when the rhythm is so totally irregular that it is unpredictable and does not follow a fixed pattern.

3. Identify and examine the P waves. Determine whether the shape is normal and note whether every P wave is followed by a QRS complex. Count the P waves to calculate the atrial rate and compare that rate to the ventricular heart rate.

4. Measure the P-R interval to determine the amount of time that elapses between the firing of the S-A node and the conduction of the impulse by the A-V node. This measurement is normally between 0.12 seconds and 0.20 seconds (3 to 5 small squares on ECG paper).

5. Measure the width of the QRS complex from the beginning of the Q wave to the end of the S wave. The normal width of

the QRS complex does not exceed 0.10 seconds (2½ small squares on ECG paper).

The importance of following these five steps when evaluating the ECG recording cannot be overemphasized. Again, stated briefly, they are:
1. Calculate the ventricular heart rate.
2. Determine the rhythm of the R waves.
3. Identify and examine the P waves.
4. Measure the P-R interval.
5. Measure the width of the QRS complex.

CLASSIFICATION OF ARRHYTHMIAS

Although there are several ways of classifying arrhythmias, the two most common methods are based on (1) the area of the heart from which they arise and (2) the physiological mechanism involved.

Classification according to area of origin:
1. *Sinoatrial node*
   Arrhythmias that originate in the S-A node are usually called "sinus." For example: sinus tachycardia, sinus bradycardia, sinus arrhythmia, and sinus arrest.
2. *Atria*
   Arrhythmias that originate in the atria are usually called "atrial." For example: premature atrial contractions, wandering atrial pacemaker (may also be classified with sinus arrhythmias), paroxysmal atrial tachycardia, atrial flutter, and atrial fibrillation.
3. *Atrioventricular junction (node)*
   Arrhythmias that originate in the atrioventricular junction are usually called "junctional" or "nodal." For example: A-V junctional (nodal) rhythms, premature

junctional (nodal) contractions and junctional (nodal) tachycardia.

Atrioventricular conduction defects also have their origin in the A-V junction and are referred to as forms of heart block. For example: first degree heart block, second degree heart block, and complete (third degree) heart block.

4. *Ventricles*
Arrhythmias that originate in the ventricles are usually called "ventricular." For example: premature ventricular contractions, ventricular tachycardia, ventricular flutter, ventricular fibrillation.

Classification according to the physiological mechanism involved:
Occasionally, arrhythmias are classified according to the related underlying clinical problem. Lown et al (1967) recommended that arrhythmias be classified as follows*:

Arrhythmia Category	Specific Disorder	Prognosis
Electrical instability	Ventricular extrasystoles Ventricular tachycardia	Good
Potential electrical instability	Sinus bradycardia Nodal extrasystoles Nodal rhythm Heart block	Excellent (except in cases of 2nd and 3rd degree heart block)
Pump failure	Sinus tachycardia Atrial extrasystoles Atrial and nodal tachycardia Atrial flutter Atrial fibrillation	Poor

* Lown, B. et al. "Unsolved problems in coronary care." *American Journal of Cardiology* 20: 498 (October, 1967).

IDENTIFICATION OF ARRHYTHMIAS

The diagram in Figure 3-1 will be used as a basis for illustrating the abnormalities of conduction that occur when arrhythmias are present.

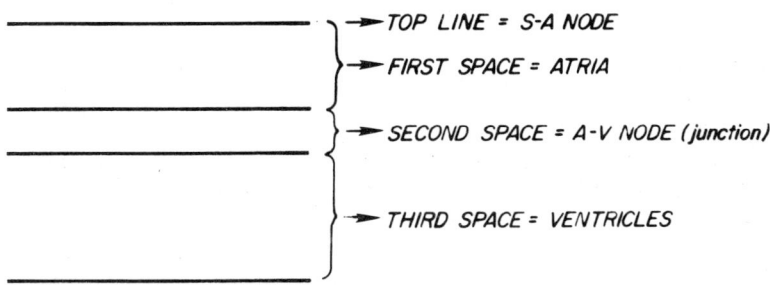

Figure 3-1. Diagram of the phases in the progression of electrical impulses through the heart.

The spaces between the lines represent the time it takes an electrical impulse to travel from its point of origin in the S-A node through the heart. As will be shown in further diagrams, these time periods vary in different arrhythmias.

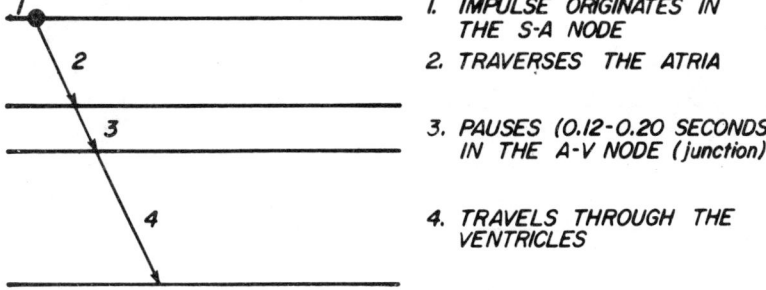

Figure 3-2. Diagram of the progression of electrical impulses in normal sinus rhythm.

Sinus Arrhythmias

In all sinus arrhythmias the impulse originates in the S-A node and travels through the conduction system along the normal route. Therefore, all sinus arrhythmias have a normal P wave and a normal QRS complex.

Sinus Tachycardia

In sinus tachycardia the S-A node maintains the pacemaking function and initiates impulses at a rate of 100 to 180 beats per minute. Some of the causes of this rapid stimulation of the S-A node are fever, pain, exercise, eating, anxiety, hemorrhage, heart disease, hypoxia, or such drugs as atropine, aminophylline, and Isuprel.

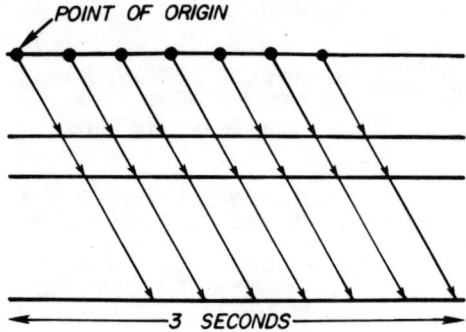

Figure 3-3. Diagram of the progression of electrical impulses in sinus tachycardia.

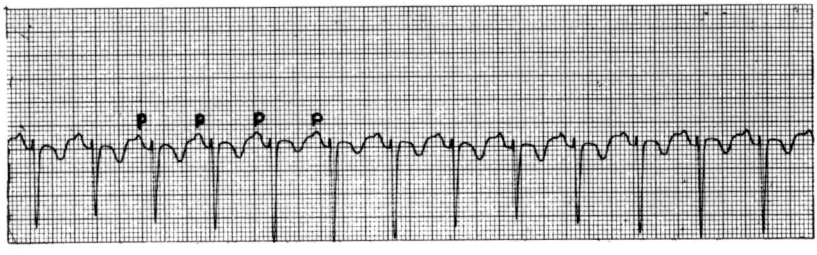

ARRHYTHMIAS

a.

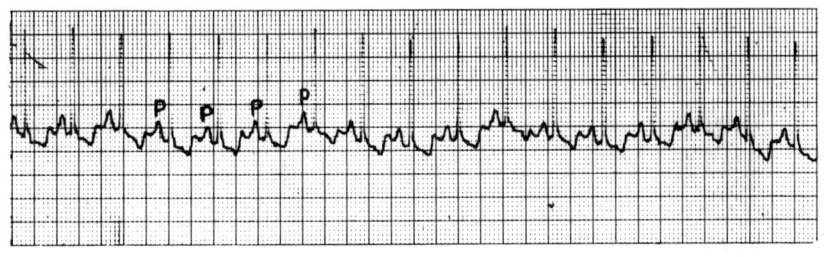

b.

Figure 3-4, a and b. Examples of the ECG in sinus tachycardia.

ECG characteristics
  Rate: 100–180
  Rhythm: Regular
  P waves: Normal; precede every QRS complex
  P-R interval: Normal
  QRS complex: Normal

Sinus Bradycardia

In sinus bradycardia the S-A node maintains its pacemaking function and initiates impulses at a rate of less than 60 beats per minute. It may be caused by vagal (parasympathetic) stimulation, digitalis or propranolol therapy, or underlying heart disease. Sinus bradycardia may also be seen in highly trained athletes.

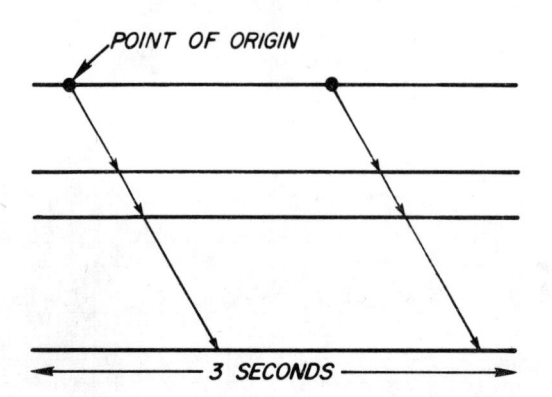

Figure 3-5. Diagram of the progression of electrical impulses in sinus bradycardia.

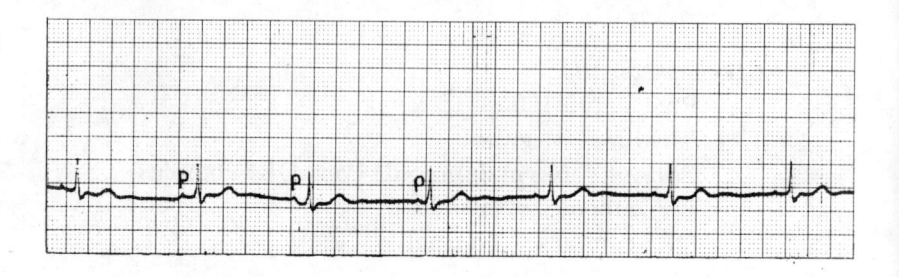

Figure 3-6. Example of the ECG in sinus bradycardia.

ECG characteristics
    Rate: Less than 60 (usually 40-60)
    Rhythm: Regular
    P waves: Normal
    P-R interval: Normal
    QRS complex: Normal

ARRHYTHMIAS

Sinus Arrhythmia

In sinus arrhythmia the impluse originates in the S-A node in a somewhat irregular rhythm. There are two varieties of sinus arrhythmia. The most common form is seen on the ECG as a change in rhythm that is related to respirations. The heart rate gradually increases on inspiration and decreases on expiration. This is considered a normal physiological variation that is seen more often in young people than adults. A less common form of sinus arrhythmia is when an irregularity in rhythm alone occurs which has no relationship to respirations or external factors. This arrhythmia may be indicative of heart disease.

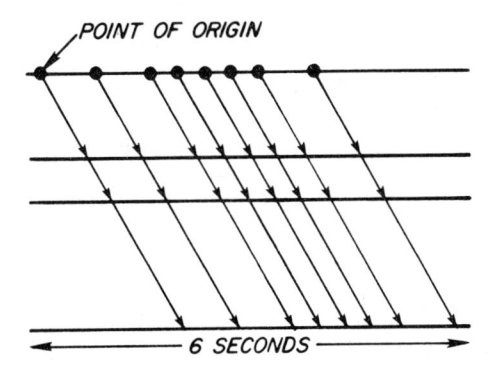

Figure 3-7. Diagram of the progression of electrical impulses in sinus arrhythmia.

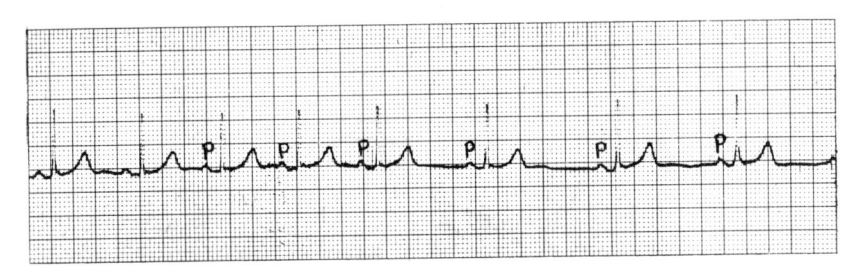

Figure 3-8. Example of the ECG in sinus arrhythmia.

ECG characteristics
    Rate: Normal (60-100) with variations related to changes in rhythm
    Rhythm: Irregular, usually related to respirations
    P waves: Normal
    P-R interval: Normal
    QRS complex: Normal

Sinus Arrest

Sinus arrest occurs when there is a pause in the rhythm due to failure of the S-A node to fire at the expected time. The duration of the pause may or may not be as long as the time required for one complete heartbeat. Sinus arrest is usually caused by increased vagal stimulation. It may also be drug induced, often as a result of digitalis toxicity, or it may be caused by organic heart disease.

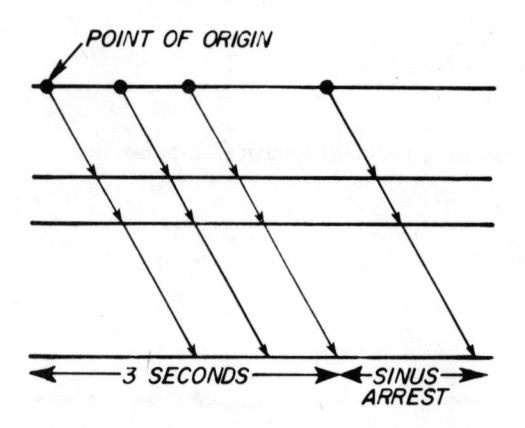

Figure 3-9. Diagram of the progression of electrical impulses in sinus arrest.

ARRHYTHMIAS

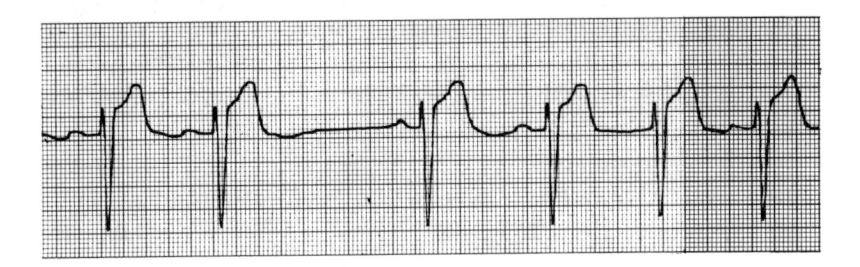

Figure 3-10. Example of the ECG in sinus arrest.

ECG characteristics
    Rate: Usually normal — may be in the range usually seen in bradycardia
    Rhythm: Normal — except for the pause caused by the absent beat
    P waves: P wave delayed due to pause in the firing of the S-A node
    P-R interval: None
    QRS complex: None

Atrial Arrhythmias

All atrial arrhythmias probably arise from an ectopic focus or circus movement within one of the atria.

Premature Atrial Contractions
(PACs; APCs)

When an ectopic focus that exists outside the S-A node (in either atrium) fires prematurely, it stimulates contraction of the atria for one or more isolated beats. The impulse travels across the atria in an abnormal fashion, creating a distorted P wave that occurs earlier than the expected beat. If the P wave is very premature and occurs during the refractory period of the ventricles it will not be followed by a QRS complex. The time interval between a PAC and the following beat is usually prolonged but is not as long as a full compensatory pause. This means that the time interval between the sinus beat that precedes the PAC and the sinus beat that follows the PAC is *not equal* to the time interval of two consecutive sinus beats. The firing of the ectopic focus in the atrium causes the sinus node to reset itself, resulting in this temporary change in rhythm.

Atrial premature beats often occur in normal individuals and may be caused by emotional disturbances or the use of tobacco, coffee, or tea. When associated with organic heart disease, they may lead to paroxysmal atrial tachycardia or atrial fibrillation.

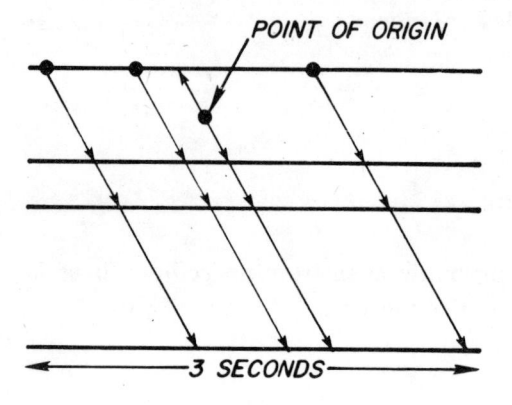

Figure 3-11. Diagram of the progression of electrical impulses in premature atrial contraction.

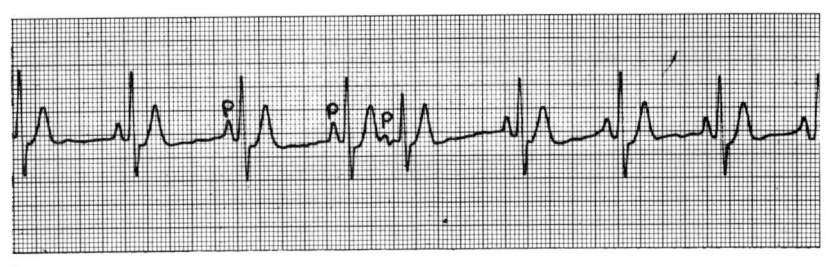

ARRHYTHMIAS

a.

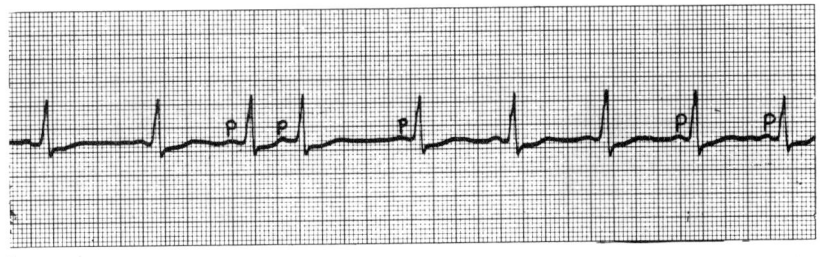

b.

Figure 3-12, a and b. Examples of the ECG in premature atrial contraction.

ECG characteristics
  Rate: Normal (60-100)
  Rhythm: Basically normal except for the occurrence of PACs
  P waves: Abnormally shaped when PACs occur
  P-R interval: Normal
  QRS complex: Normal

Wandering Atrial Pacemaker

Sometimes there will be a continued change in the location of the heart's pacemaker. It wanders within the S-A node, from the S-A node to the A-V node, or to various foci throughout the atria. The size and shape of the P-R interval may also be variable. Wandering of the atrial pacemaker is probably caused by increased vagal stimulation, but it may also result from digitalis therapy or from organic heart disease.

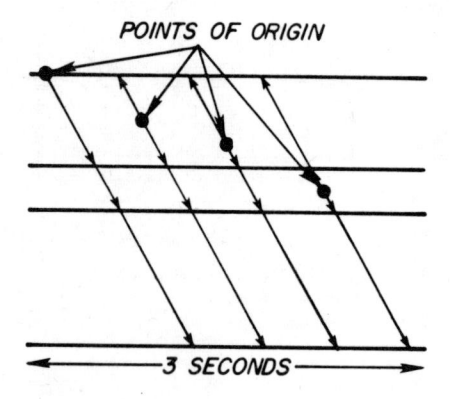

Figure 3-13. Diagram of the progression of electrical impulses when a wandering atrial pacemaker exists.

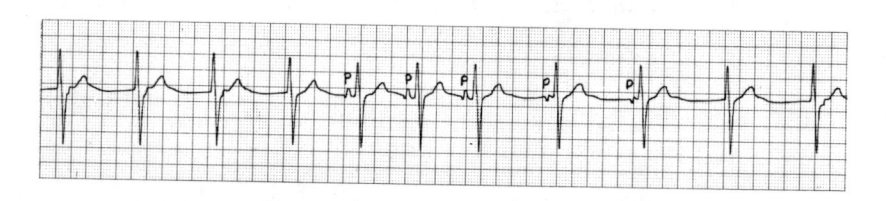

Figure 3-14. Example of the ECG when a wandering atrial pacemaker exists.

ECG characteristics
    Rate: Normal
    Rhythm: Normal
    P waves: Present: shape varies as the pacemaker wanders
    P-R interval: From the A-V node downward conduction is normal; above the A-V node conduction depends on the site of origin of the impulse
    QRS complex: Normal

Paroxysmal Atrial Tachycardia (PAT)

When an ectopic focus within the atria becomes the pacemaker, impulses are initiated at a rate of 160 to 250 beats per minute. Paroxysmal atrial tachycardia (PAT) is the term used to describe a continuous run of premature atrial contractions. The onset and termination of PAT are often abrupt. It commonly occurs in normal individuals and is often caused by emotional trauma. It may be associated with mitral valve disease, coronary artery disease, or thyrotoxicosis.

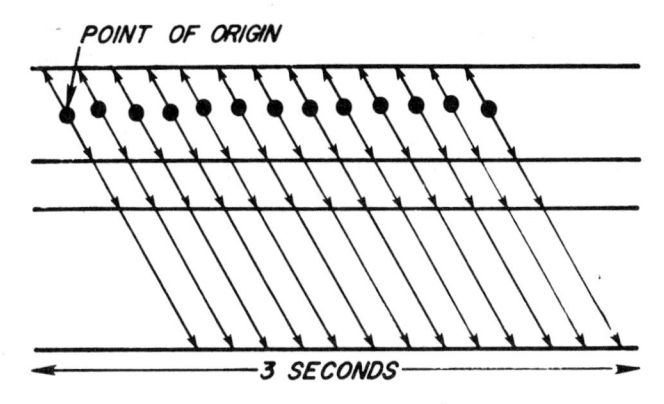

Figure 3-15. Diagram of the progression of electrical impulses in paroxysmal atrial tachycardia.

a.

b.

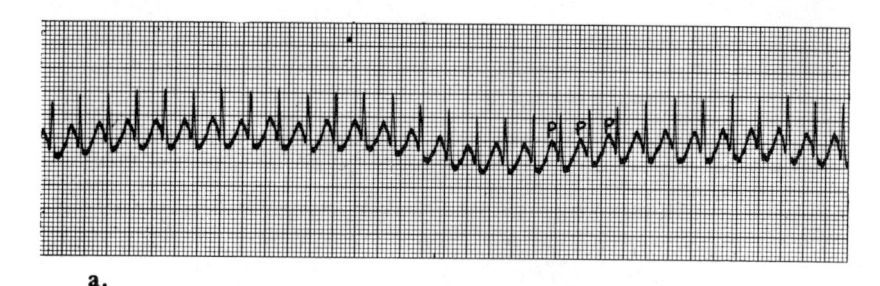

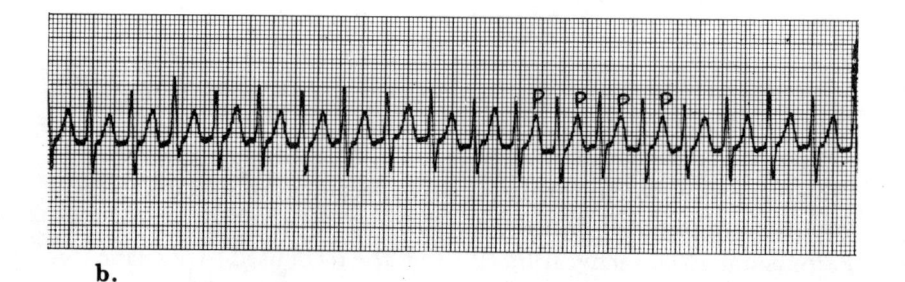

Figure 3-16, a and b. Examples of the ECG in paroxysmal atrial tachycardia.

ECG characteristics
    Rate: 160-250
    Rhythm: Regular
    P waves: Abnormally shaped; may be buried in preceding QRS complex or T wave
    P-R interval: May be prolonged
    QRS complex: Normal

Atrial Flutter

Atrial flutter occurs when an ectopic focus within the atrium initiates impulses at a rate of 220 to 350 beats per minute. It is

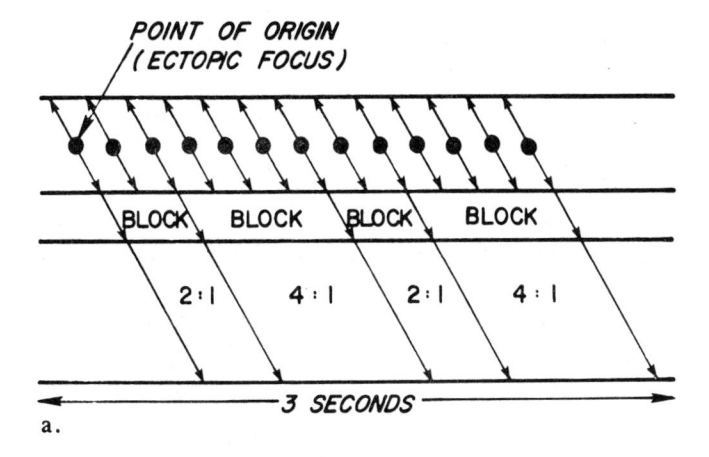

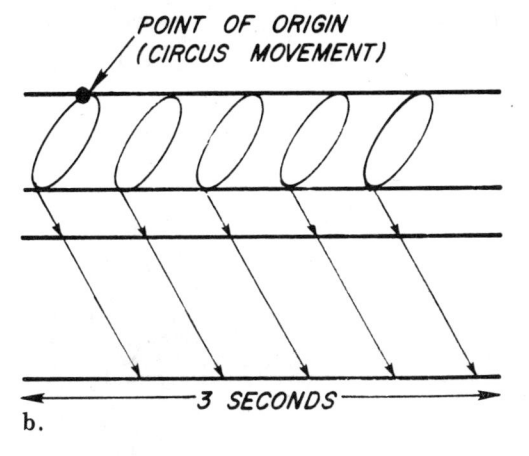

Figure 3-17, a and b. Diagrams of the progression of electrical impulses in atrial flutter. a. Atrial flutter in which a single ectopic focus in the atrium gives rise to impulses at a rate of 220 to 350 beats per minute. b. Atrial flutter in which a circus movement in the atrium gives rise to electrical impulses.

thought by some that a single ectopic focus in the atrium stimulates atrial depolarization; others believe that atrial flutter arises from a "circus" movement in the atria. It is also claimed by some that atrial flutter cannot be differentiated from paroxysmal atrial tachycardia, and they refer to both conditions as "supraventricular tachycardia" (i.e., tachycardia originating above the ventricles), while others describe these two conditions as separate entities.

In atrial flutter the atrial rate is characterized by P waves that are saw-toothed in appearance and are often called flutter waves. An atrioventricular (A-V) block exists when there is a ratio of two or more atrial beats to one ventricular beat. A 2:1 or 4:1 ratio is most common; however, ratios of 3:1, 5:1, or 6:1 may also occur.

a.

b.

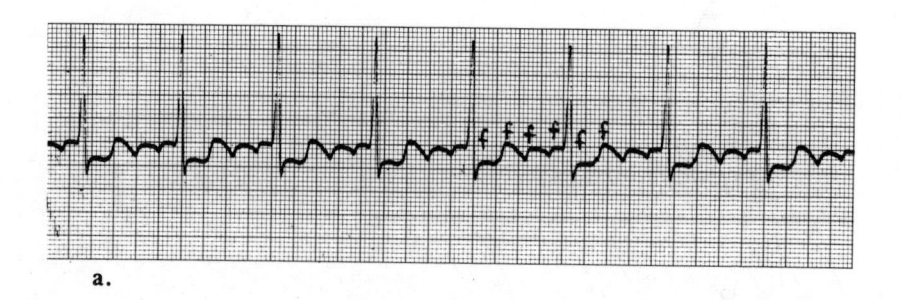

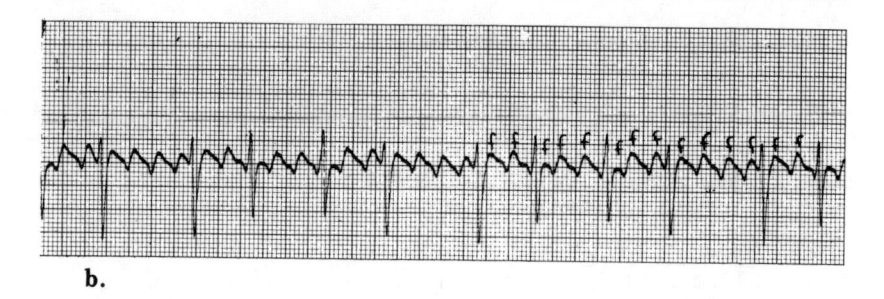

Figure 3-18, a and b. Examples of the ECG in atrial flutter.

ECG characteristics
    Rate: Atrial rate — 220 to 350
          Ventricular rate varies, depending on atrial rate and degree of A-V block
    Rhythm: Atrial rhythm regular
          Ventricular rhythm most often regular but will be irregular if a varying degree of A-V block is present
    P wave: Characteristic saw-toothed flutter waves
    P-R interval: Normal for beats conducted through the A-V node
    QRS complex: Normal

Although atrial flutter may occur in normal individuals, it is usually caused by organic heart disease. It is often seen when quinidine therapy is given to convert atrial fibrillation prior to elective cardioversion.

Atrial Fibrillation

When one of several ectopic foci within the atria discharges between 350 and 500 beats per minute atrial fibrillation results. The circus movement theory is also applied to atrial fibrillation; however, it is thought that, in this case, there are several circus movements, not just one as in atrial flutter. A chaotic, asynchronous beating of the atria creates a total effect that resembles a twitching rather than a contraction. The ventricular response (60–140 beats per minute) results in a totally irregular rhythm.
    Atrial fibrillation may occur in normal individuals but is usually caused by heart disease. It is frequently associated with disease of the mitral valve.

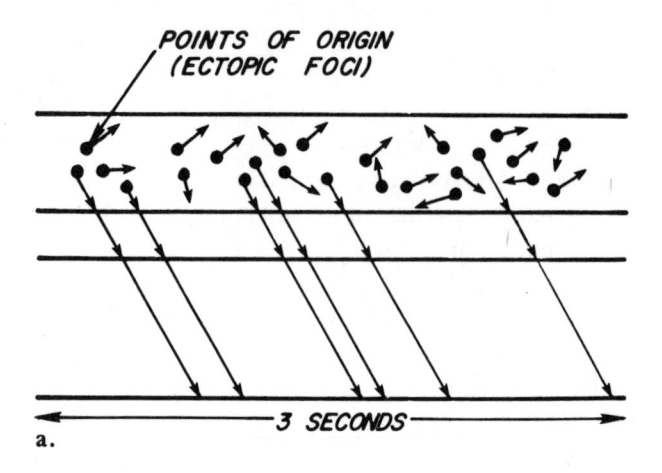

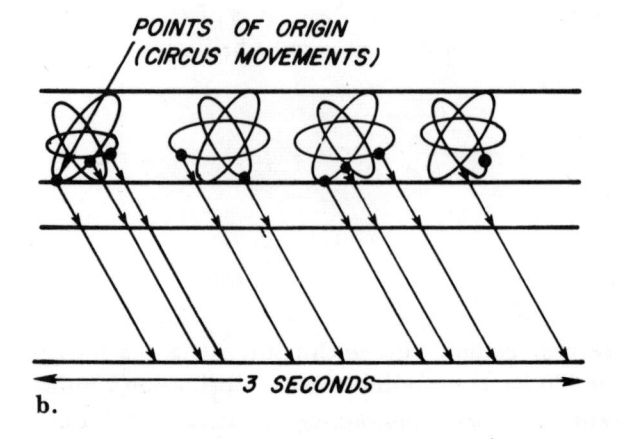

Figure 3-19, a and b. Diagrams of the progression of electrical impulses in atrial fibrillation. a. Electrical impulses arise in several ectopic foci in the atrium. b. Circus movements in the atrium give rise to electrical impulses.

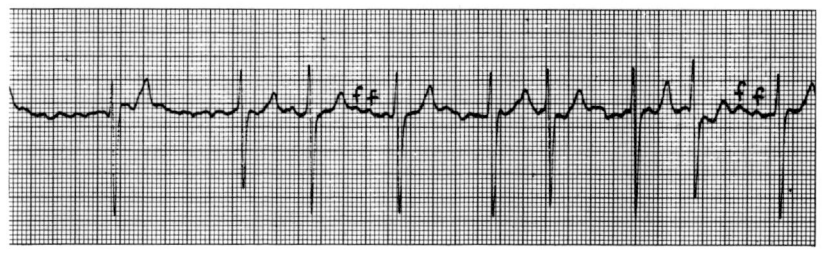

ARRHYTHMIAS

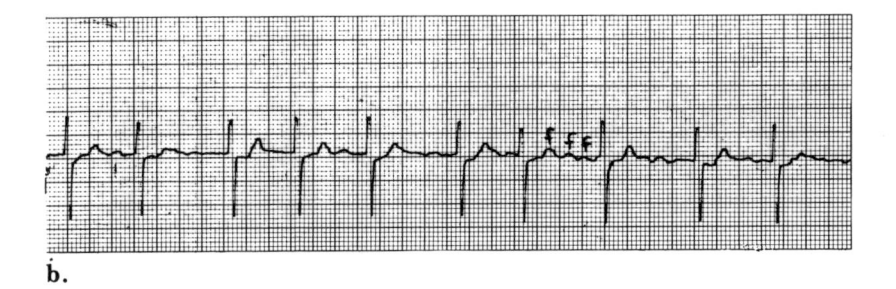

Figure 3-20, a and b. Examples of the ECG in atrial fibrillation.

ECG characteristics
    Rate: Variable; in controlled atrial fibrillation the ventricular rate is less than 100
    Rhythm: Totally irregular
    P wave: No true P waves; small irregular "f" waves
    P-R interval: Not identifiable
    QRS complex: Normal

Atrial Flutter-Fibrillation

Occasionally, fibrillation waves appear coarse and resemble flutter waves. When this occurs, the rhythm may still be called atrial fibrillation; however, other terms in use for this condition are: atrial flutter-fibrillation, impulse flutter, and coarse fibrillation.

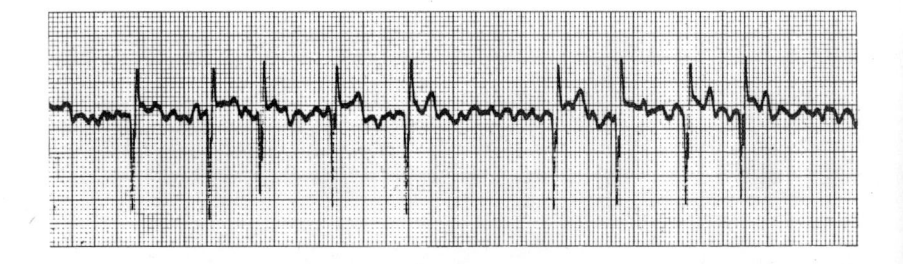

Figure 3-21. Example of the ECG in atrial flutter-fibrillation (coarse fibrillation).

Junctional (Nodal) Arrhythmias

A-V junctional (nodal) arrhythmias arise from ectopic foci in the area of the A-V junction where the A-V node and common atrioventricular bundle (bundle of His) are located. The impulse travels upward through the atria in a retrograde fashion and down through the ventricles at approximately the same time. In such rhythms the ventricular rate usually varies from 40 to 65 beats per minute with a regular ventricular rhythm. Junctional rhythms may be transient or permanent. Although they can occur in normal individuals, they may also result from organic heart disease, or they may be drug induced.

In junctional rhythms the P wave is either inverted before or after the QRS complex or may be buried within it. In the past it was believed that the origin of these arrhythmias was the A-V node and that the origin of the impulse that produces the P wave was either high in this node, in the middle of it, or in the lower part of it. Modern electrocardiographic techniques have shown that these arrhythmias originate in the junctional tissue in the area of the A-V node and bundle of His. The correct term for describing these arrhythmias is "junctional"; however, the term "nodal" is still used quite extensively.

ECG characteristics in Junctional (Nodal) Arrhythmias
    Rate: 40-65 (120-200 if tachycardia is present)
    Rhythm: Regular
    P waves: Abnormal; inverted before QRS complex, buried in QRS complex, or inverted following QRS complex
    P-R interval: Variable

        Note: When the P wave is inverted before the QRS complex, the P-R interval is usually less than 0.11 seconds. If it is longer than 0.11 seconds, the origin of the beat may be in the lower portion of the right atrium. When the P wave is buried in the QRS complex or is inverted following it, the P-R interval cannot be identified

    QRS complex: Normal
        May be distorted when the P wave is buried in it

Arrhythmias That Originate High in the A-V Junctional Area

When the ectopic focus is located in the upper portion of the A-V junctional area, the impulse spreads through the atria before reaching the ventricles. Because of retrograde conduction, the P wave is inverted and precedes the QRS complex. The P-R interval may be shorter than normal.

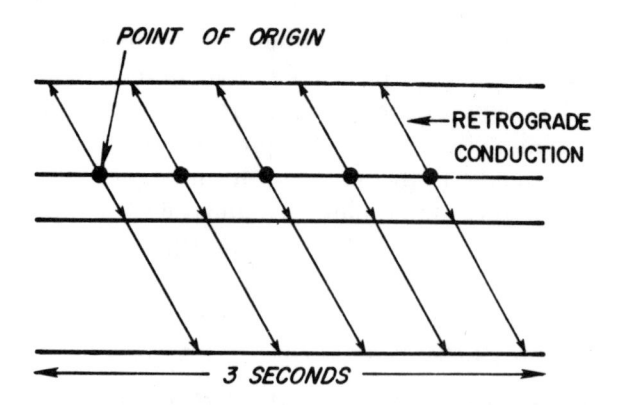

Figure 3-22. Diagram of the progression of electrical impulses in high A-V junctional rhythm.

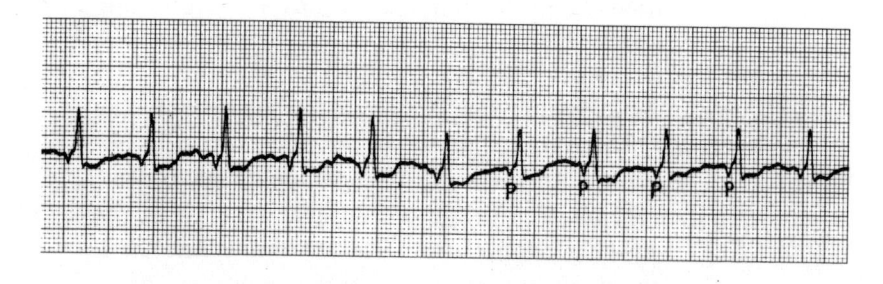

Figure 3-23. Example of the ECG in arrhythmias that originate high in the A-V junctional area.

Arrhythmias That Originate in the Middle of the A-V Junctional Area

When the ectopic focus is in the middle of the A-V junctional area, the impulse spreads through the atria and ventricles simultaneously. The P wave is buried in the QRS complex and is either unidentifiable or is seen as a notch in the QRS complex.

ARRHYTHMIAS

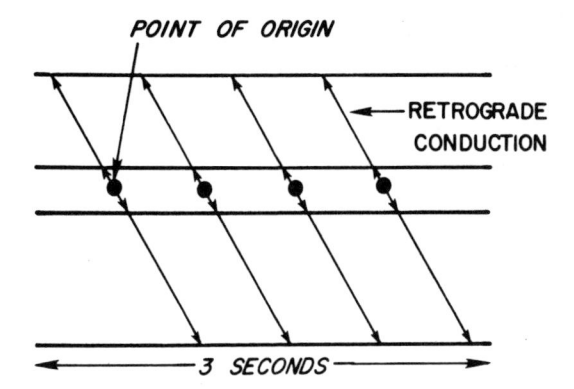

Figure 3-24. Diagram of the progression of electrical impulses in mid A-V junctional rhythm.

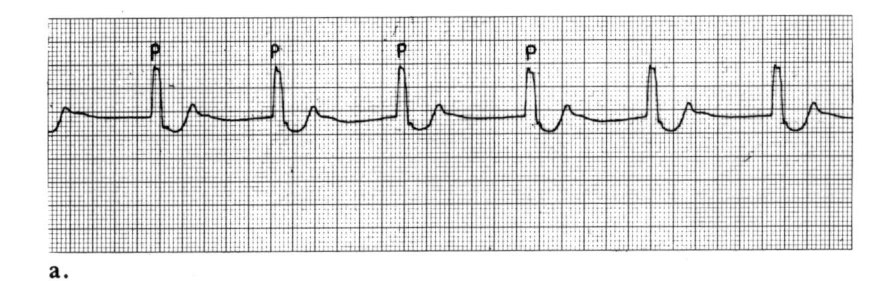

Figure 3-25, a and b. Examples of midjunctional arrhythmias in which the P waves are buried within the QRS complexes.

Rhythms That Originate Low in the A-V Junctional Area

When the impulse originates low in the A-V junctional area, the ventricles are stimulated before the atria. The QRS complex occurs first, followed closely by an inverted P wave that represents the retrograde atrial conduction.

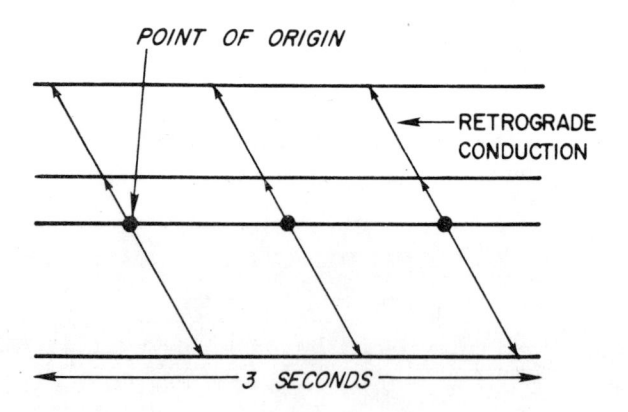

Figure 3-26. Diagram of the progression of electrical impulses in low A-V junctional rhythm.

Premature Junctional (Nodal) Contraction (PJCs, PNCs)

An ectopic focus in the A-V junctional area may become the pacemaker for occasional isolated beats. This focus may be located in the upper, middle, or lower portion of the A-V junction. The conduction and ECG pattern for these beats are the same as those described for junctional rhythms; however, this isolated beat does not constitute the primary rhythm. Although it occurs prematurely, it is not followed by a full compensatory pause.

ARRHYTHMIAS

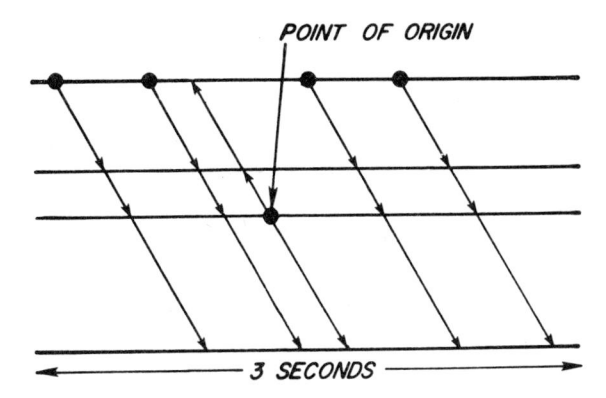

Figure 3-27. Diagram of the progression of electrical impulses in premature junctional (nodal) contractions.

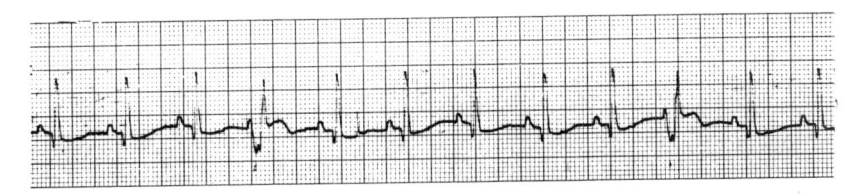

Figure 3-28. Example of the ECG in premature midjunctional contractions. Note that the fourth and tenth beats are premature contractions in which the P wave is buried within the QRS complex. The basic rhythm is normal sinus rhythm.

ECG characteristics
    Rate: Normal
    Rhythm: Basically regular except for occurrence of premature beat
    P waves: May be inverted before QRS complex, buried in QRS complex, or inverted following QRS complex
    P-R interval: Normal
        May vary with occurrence of premature beat
    QRS complex: Normal
        May appear distorted in midjunctional beat

Junctional Tachycardia

Junctional tachycardia occurs when the A-V junctional tissue becomes irritated and takes over as the heart's primary pacemaker, pacing the heart at a rate of 120 to 200 beats per minute. The fast rate often makes it difficult to differentiate this rhythm from atrial tachycardia, in which case the term supraventricular tachycardia should be used.

The characteristics of junctional tachycardias are the same as those described for junctional arrhythmias with the exception of the ventricular rate, which is in the usual range for a tachycardia.

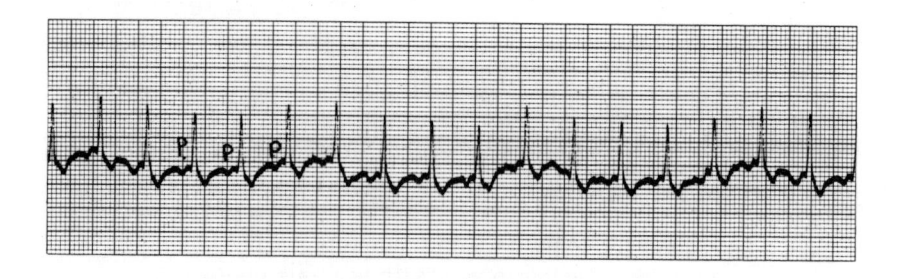

Figure 3-29. Example of the ECG in junctional tachycardia. Note that the P waves are inverted before the QRS complex.

Ventricular Arrhythmias

Ventricular arrhythmias arise from ectopic foci located in the ventricles.

Premature Ventricular Contractions
(PVCs; VPCs; VPBs)

One or more ectopic foci in the ventricles may stimulate ventricular contraction for occasional isolated premature beats. This

ARRHYTHMIAS

impulse travels through the ventricles in an abnormal fashion to produce PVC configurations that vary depending on their point of origin; however, they all have similar characteristics:
1. The duration of the QRS complex is greater than 0.12 seconds, is wide and bizarre in configuration, and appears "slurred."
2. The T wave is usually in the opposite direction from the QRS complex.
3. The PVC occurs prematurely; that is, before the time at which the normal beat would occur.
4. The PVC is followed by a full compensatory pause. The time between the beat preceding the PVC and the beat following the PVC is equal to the time between two normal R-R intervals.
5. The PVC is not preceded by a P wave. The S-A node usually fires in rhythm, but the P wave is buried in the premature QRS complex.

PVCs may occur in normal individuals and have no clinical significance. Organic heart disease (congestive heart failure, myocardial infarction, etc.) is a common cause of PVCs. Although they may be controlled with digitalis therapy, premature ventricular contractions may also be one of the symptoms of digitalis toxicity.

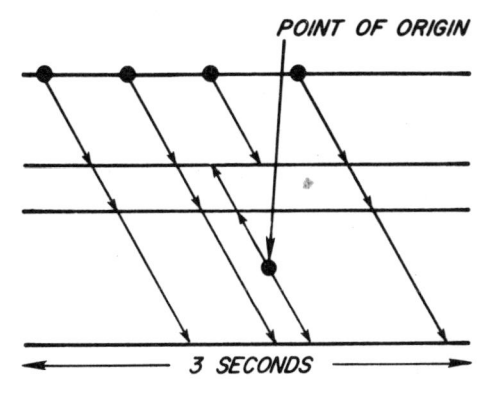

Figure 3-30. Diagram of the progression of electrical impulses in premature ventricular contractions.

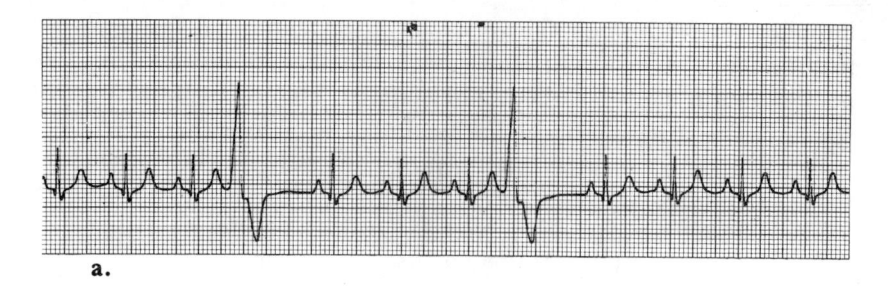

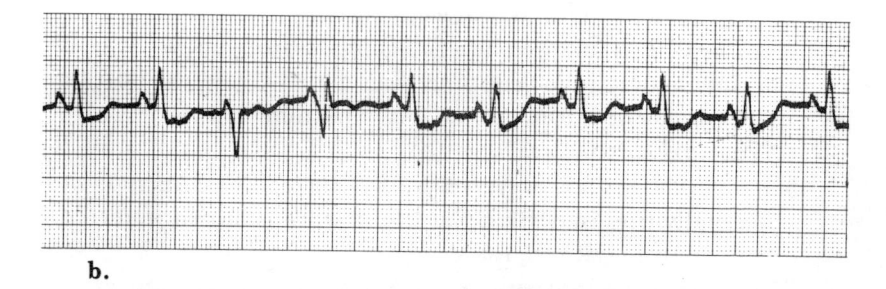

Figure 3-31, a and b. Examples of the ECG in premature ventricular contractions. Note that in the first strip the fourth and eighth beats are PVCs. In the second strip the third and fourth beats are PVCs. In both instances the basic rhythm is normal sinus rhythm.

ECG characteristics

- Rate: Normal
- Rhythm: The time between the beats preceding and following the PVC is equal to the normal time for two beats
- P waves: Present, but usually buried in the QRS complex
- P-R interval: No conduction between atria and ventricles for isolated PVC
- QRS complex: Slurred and widened (width greater than 0.12 seconds)

ARRHYTHMIAS

Bigeminy (Coupled Rhythm)

In bigeminy every other beat is a PVC that usually alternates with a normal beat. The interval between the sinus beat and the premature beat is usually constant (fixed coupling). Occasionally the PVC couples with an atrial or junctional (nodal) beat.

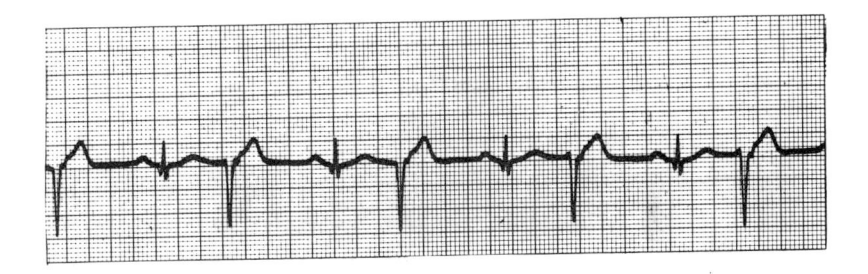

Figure 3-32. Example of the ECG in bigeminy. Note that each normal sinus beat is followed by a PVC.

Trigeminy (Trigeminal Rhythm)

In trigeminy every third beat is a PVC, *or* every sinus beat is followed by two PVCs.

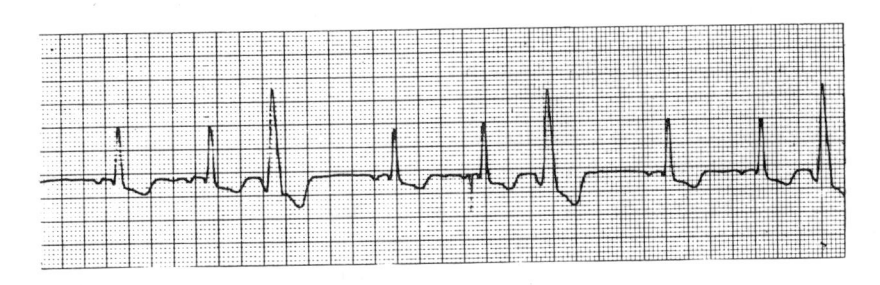

Figure 3-33. Example of the ECG in trigeminy. Note that every two normal sinus beats are followed by a PVC.

Additional Notes on PVCs

Interpolated PVCs: A PVC falls between two normal beats and *is not* followed by a compensatory pause. This may occur when the ventricular focus fires so prematurely that the ventricles are able to respond to the next sinus impulse.

Unifocal PVCs: All PVCs recorded on the same lead have the same configuration and therefore arise from the same ectopic focus.

Multifocal PVCs: PVCs recorded on the same lead have different configurations, indicating that they arise from different ectopic foci. This condition indicates a high degree of myocardial irritability.

Multiform Unifocal PVCs: This term is applied to ventricular beats that have different configurations of the QRS complex but have a constant R-R interval. This indicates that they are from the same focus but follow a different pathway through the ventricles.

Ventricular Tachycardia (VT)

Ventricular tachycardia is present when three or more PVCs occur in a row. It occurs when an ectopic focus in the ventricles fires at a rate of 140 to 220 beats per minute. The rhythm is often slightly irregular. Ventricular tachycardia is a serious arrhythmia and is almost always associated with serious organic heart disease or drug toxicity. On rare occasions, it is seen in normal individuals.

ARRHYTHMIAS

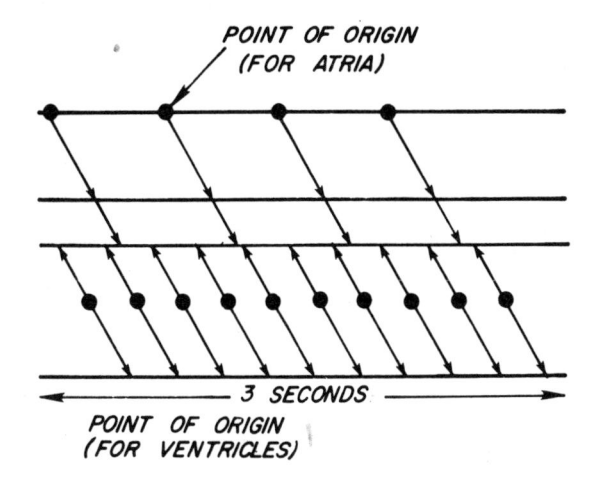

Figure 3-34. Diagram of the progression of electrical impulses in ventricular tachycardia.

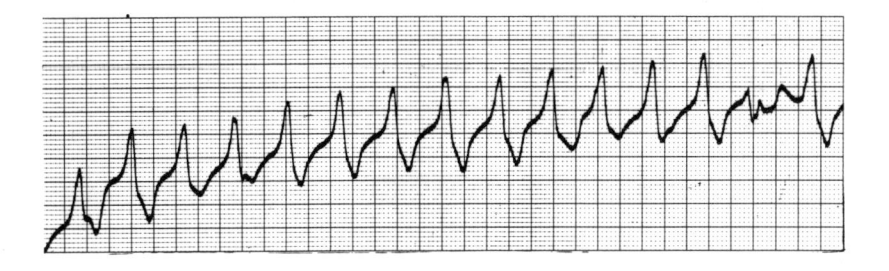

Figure 3-35. Example of the ECG in ventricular tachycardia.

ECG characteristics

    Rate: Usually 140-220

    Rhythm: Slightly irregular

    P waves: Usually present but buried in the QRS complex

    P-R interval: Unidentifiable—atria and ventricles beat independently of each other

    QRS complex: Bizarre—widened and slurred (resembles the QRS complex in PVC)

Additional Notes about Ventricular Tachycardia

In ventricular tachycardia, if the S-A node is still firing, P waves will occur but they are frequently buried in the QRS complex, occasionally appearing as a notch in it. It is often difficult to distinguish ventricular tachycardia from supraventricular tachycardia, particularly when the latter occurs with a bundle branch block or aberrant conduction. When there is a bundle branch block, i.e., an obstruction in one of the bundle branches, depolarization of the affected ventricle is delayed and the QRS complex becomes distorted. In aberrant conduction, the impulse that has entered the ventricle through the A-V node and bundle of His wanders from the normal pathway, resulting in abnormal depolarization of the ventricle and a distorted QRS complex:

Occasionally, there is a ventricular rhythm with a rate as low as 70. Although this is not ventricular tachycardia by definition, the physiological abnormality is the same and it is sometimes referred to as ventricular tachycardia.

Ventricular Flutter

This term is often used to describe a rapid ventricular tachycardia in which the QRS complexes are large wave-like oscillations.

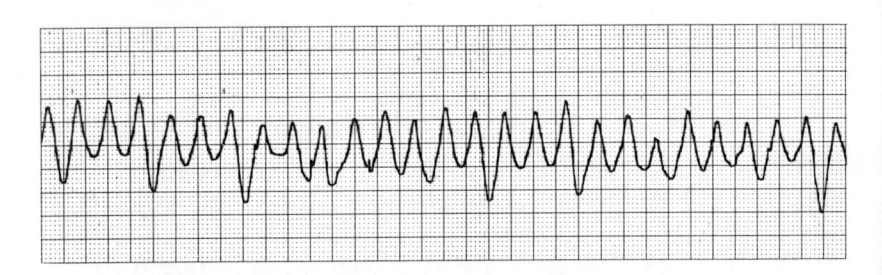

Figure 3-36. Example of the ECG in ventricular flutter.

Ventricular Fibrillation

When one (or more) foci within the ventricles fires at a very rapid rate the ventricular muscle is unable to respond. This results in twitching of the ventricles. The ventricular complexes are rapid, irregular, and bizarre, with no identifiable P waves, QRS complexes, or T waves. This is the most serious arrhythmia and will terminate in cardiac standstill if not treated immediately.

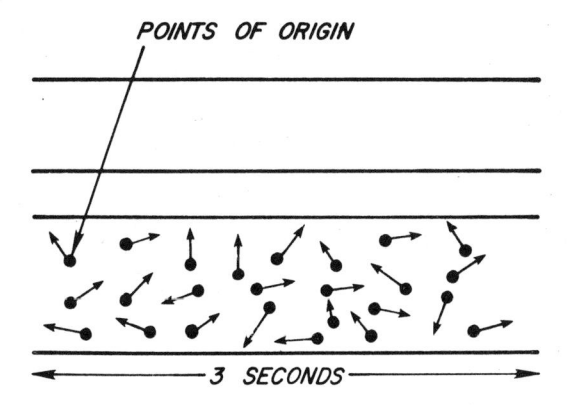

Figure 3-37. Diagram of the progression of electrical impulses in ventricular fibrillation.

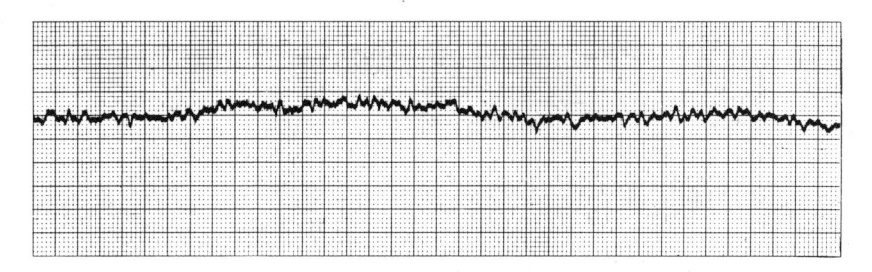

Figure 3-38. Example of the ECG in ventricular fibrillation.

CONDUCTION DEFECTS

A conduction defect exists when impulses that arise in the atria are not conducted through the A-V junction (node) to the ventricles at the normal rate (0.12 to 0.20 seconds). The disturbance in conduction may be partial (incomplete) or complete and result in partial or complete heart block.

First Degree Heart Block

When the conduction of the impulse through the A-V junction is delayed longer than 0.20 seconds, first degree heart block is present. Every impulse is conducted through the A-V junction; the length of the P-R interval remains constant; and every P wave is followed by a QRS complex.

First degree heart block may occur in the presence of many infectious diseases or organic heart disease, or it may result from drug intoxication (especially digitalis).

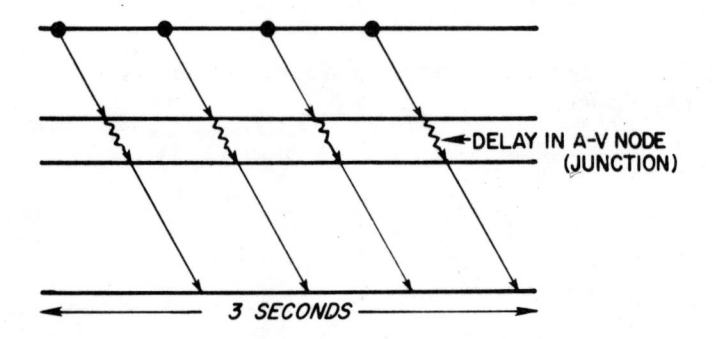

Figure 3-39. Diagram of the progression of electrical impulses in first degree heart block.

ARRHYTHMIAS

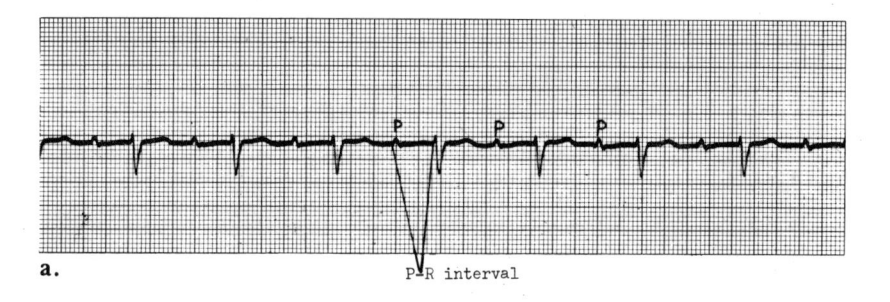

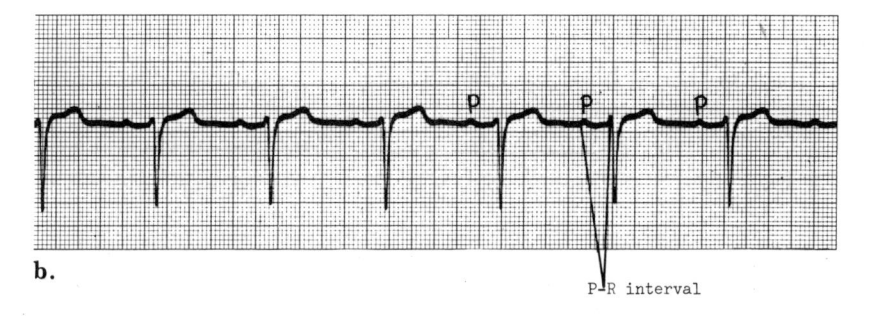

Figure 3-40, a and b. Examples of the ECG in first degree heart block.

ECG characteristics
    Rate: Normal
    Rhythm: Regular
    P waves: Normal
    P-R interval: Prolonged beyond 0.20 seconds
    QRS complex: Normal

Second Degree Heart Block

When the A-V junction conducts some, but not all, of the impulses originating in the atria, second degree heart block is present. The number of nonconducted (or dropped) beats varies, depending on the degree of block that exists. The atrial rate is always greater than the ventricular rate. Second degree heart block may be due to organic (cardiac) disease or to digitalis toxicity.

In second degree heart block there may be an occasional nonconducted beat. For example, there may be eight P waves for every seven QRS complexes; this is called an 8:7 block.

In severe A-V block, the A-V junction conducts fewer beats. For example, there may be four P waves for every QRS complex; this is called a 4:1 block. Although the degree of block often remains the same, there may be a constant change in conduction. For example, conduction may change so that the block varies from a 2:1 block to a 4:1 A-V block. A first degree A-V block (prolonged P-R interval) is occasionally seen with the conducted beats.

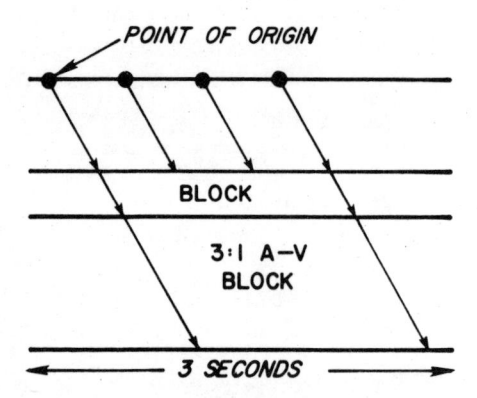

Figure 3-41. Diagram of the progression of electrical impulses in second degree A-V block.

ARRHYTHMIAS

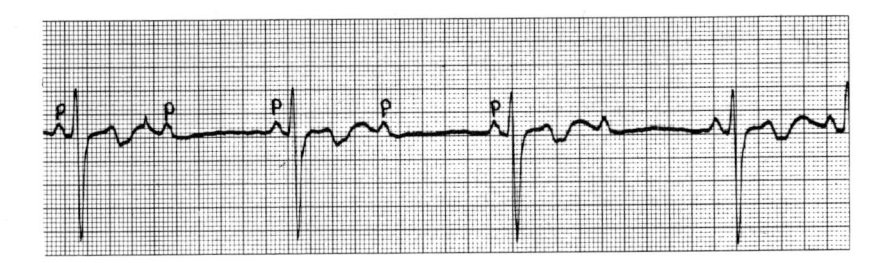

Figure 3-42. Example of the ECG in second degree heart block.

ECG characteristics

Rate: Ventricular rate is usually slow and is less than the atrial rate

Rhythm: Usually regular but may be irregular if a varying degree of block is present

P waves: Normal

P-R interval: May be normal or prolonged for conducted beats. Absent for nonconducted beats

QRS complex: Normal

Additional Note about Second Degree Heart Block

Wenckeback Phenomenon (Mobitz I): In this phenomenon there is a gradual prolongation of the P-R interval (an increase in degree of A-V block) until one beat is not conducted (dropped). Usually the P-R interval of the first beat in the cycle is normal and shorter that that of all beats following it. The number of beats in each cycle may vary.

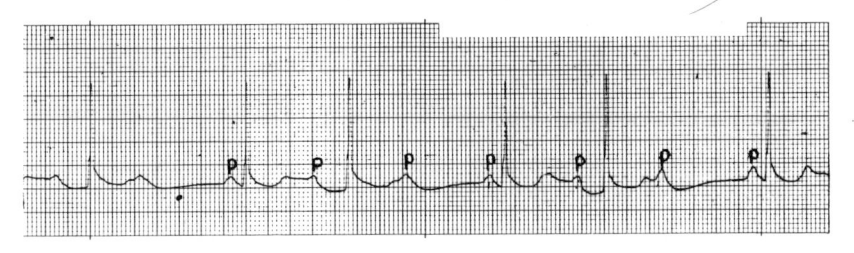

Figure 3-43. Example of the ECG in the Wenckeback phenomenon (also called Mobitz I block).

Complete Heart Block (Third Degree)

When the A-V junction does not conduct any impulses from the atria, complete heart block exists and the atria and ventricles beat independently of each other. The S-A node continues to pace the atria at a normal rate while the ventricles beat at a much slower rate in response to an ectopic focus that arises below the site of the block. Although the P waves and QRS complexes occur regularly, they have no relationship to each other. Occasionally, a P wave may fall before a QRS complex, giving the appearance of a normally conducted beat; However, this is just a coincidence and does *not* indicate a conducted beat.

Complete heart block may occur when organic (cardiac) heart disease is present, or it may be due to digitalis toxicity.

In complete heart block, the shape of the QRS complex varies according to its site of origin. If the focus is in the A-V junction, or high in the common bundle, the QRS complex may have a normal appearance and the ventricular rate will be between 40 and 55 beats per minute. The lower the focus is in the ventricles, the more bizarre the QRS complex will appear.

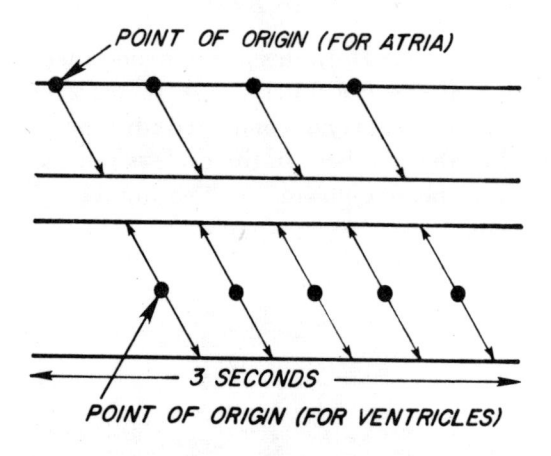

Figure 3-44. Diagram of the progression of electrical impulses in complete heart block.

ARRHYTHMIAS

Occasionally, more than one focus paces the ventricles. This increases the ventricular rate, causes the appearance of QRS complexes of differing configurations, and may result in an irregular ventricular rhythm.

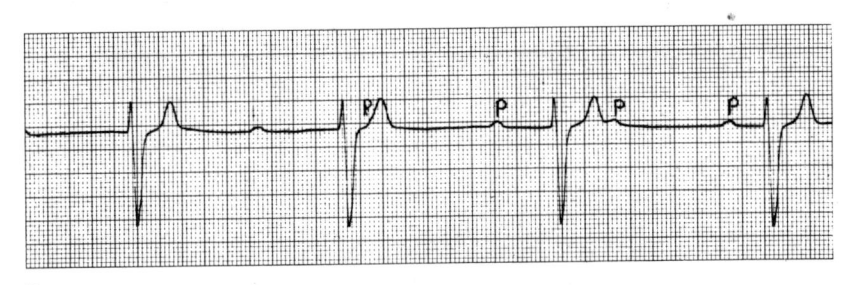

a.

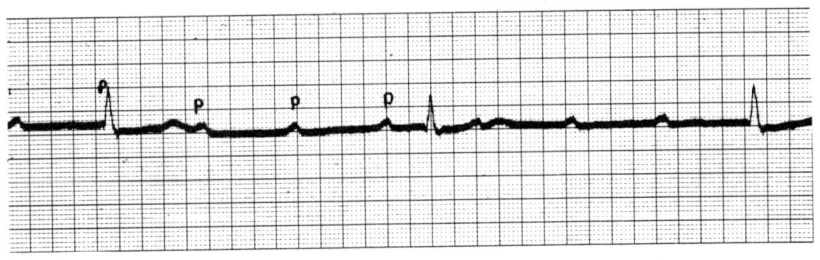

b.

Figure 3-45, a and b. Examples of the ECG in complete heart block.

ECG characteristics
- Rate: Ventricular rate usually 20-40; atrial rate usually normal (60-100)
- Rhythm: Atrial rhythm normal
  Ventricular rhythm usually normal
- P waves: Normal but some may be buried in QRS
- P-R interval: Absent—the atria and ventricles beat independently of each other
- QRS complex: Usually abnormal, depending on the site of the focus that is causing ventricular stimulation

SOME SAMPLE RHYTHM STRIPS

The following rhythm strips demonstrate basic arrhythmias. In several instances more than one arrhythmia occurs, and this makes these strips somewhat more difficult to evaluate.

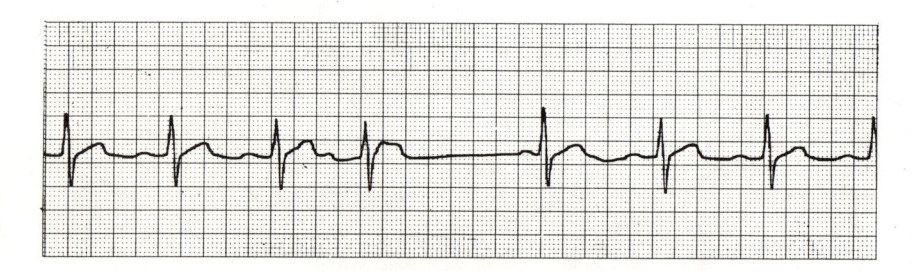

Figure 3-46. Normal sinus rhythm; PAC followed by sinus arrest.

    Rate: 65, except between beats 3 to 5
    Rhythm: Regular, except between beats 3 to 5
    P waves: Present, except for a long pause following the fourth beat
    P-R interval: 0.28 seconds (prolonged)
    QRS complex: Normal, except for a long pause following the fourth beat
    Arrhythmia present: Basic rhythm is first degree heart block
        The fourth beat is a premature atrial contraction followed by sinus pause

ARRHYTHMIAS

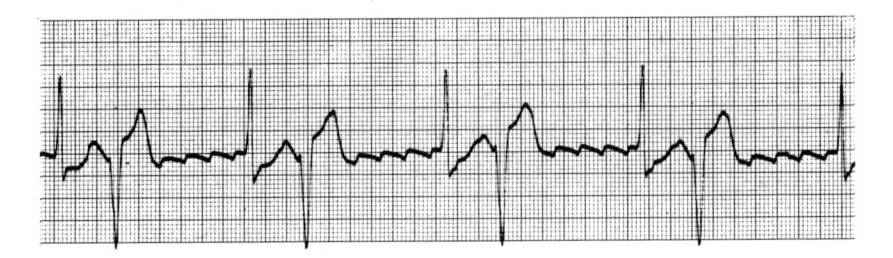

Figure 3-47. Atrial flutter with ventricular bigeminy.

Rate: Atrial 250; ventricular 65
Rhythm: Regular-irregular
P waves: Absent; saw-toothed flutter waves present
P-R interval: Unidentifiable
QRS complex: Every normal complex is followed by a QRS complex that appears widened and slurred
Arrhythmia present: Atrial flutter with an 8:1 block and ventricular bigeminy (every other QRS complex is a PVC)

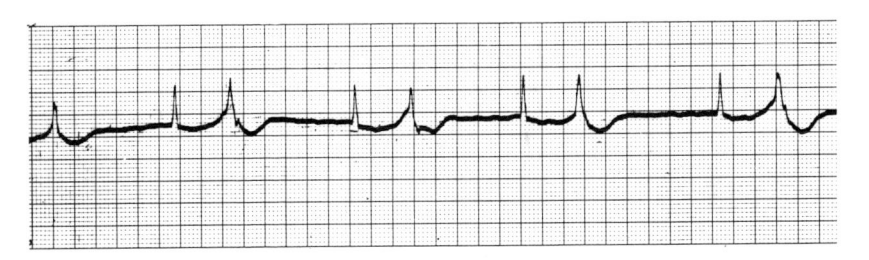

Figure 3-48. Atrial fibrillation with ventricular bigeminy.

Rate: 70-80
Rhythm: Irregular
P waves: Absent; fibrillation waves are present
P-R interval: Unidentifiable
QRS complex: Every normal QRS complex is followed by a QRS complex that appears widened and slurred
Arrhythmia present: Atrial fibrillation with ventricular bigeminy

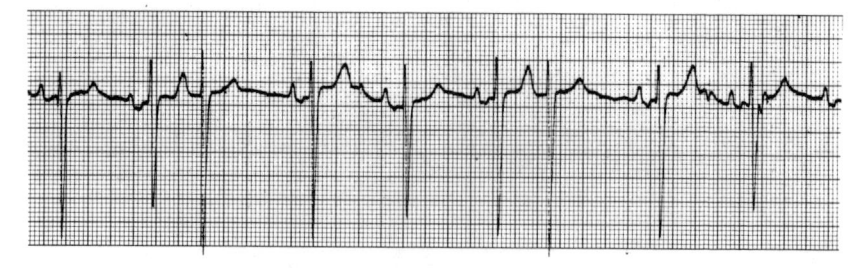

Figure 3-49. Atrial quadrigeminy. Every fourth beat is a PAC.

Rate: Approximately 80
Rhythm: Regular—irregular
P waves: Present; every fourth P wave is buried in the preceding QRS complex
P-R interval: 0.18 seconds (normal)
Arrhythmia present: Atrial quadrigeminy; normal sinus rhythm; every fourth beat is a PAC

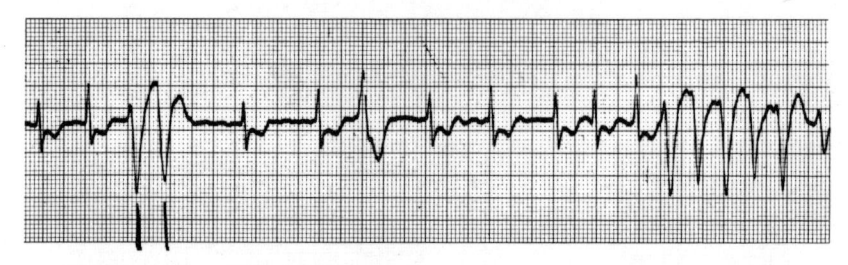

Figure 3-50. Atrial fibrillation with short runs of ventricular tachycardia.

Rate: Approximately 120
Rhythm: Irregular
P waves: Absent; fibrillation waves are present
P-R interval: Unidentifiable
QRS complex: Normal except for the third, fourth, seventh, thirteenth, fourteenth, fifteenth, sixteenth, and seventeenth complexes which are widened and slurred
Arrhythmia present: Atrial fibrillation with short runs of ventricular tachycardia

ARRHYTHMIAS

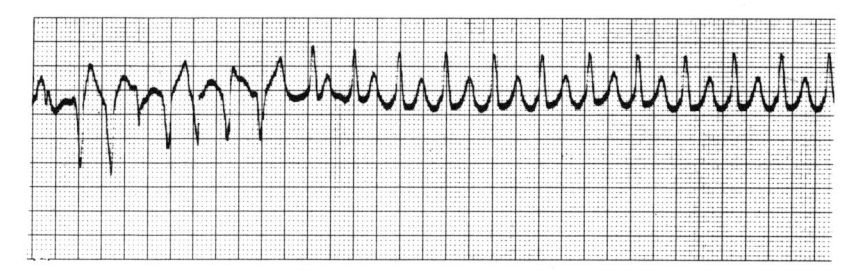

Figure 3-51. Ventricular tachycardia followed by paroxysmal atrial tachycardia.

    Rate: On the first third of the strip the rate is 250; on the last two-thirds of the strip it is 150
    Rhythm: Regular on both sections of strip
    P waves: Unidentifiable; probably buried in the T waves on the last two-thirds of the strip
    P-R interval: Unidentifiable
    QRS complex: Widened and slurred on the first third of the strip; normal on the last two-thirds of the strip
    Arrhythmia present: Ventricular tachycardia followed by paroxysmal atrial tachycardia (PAT)

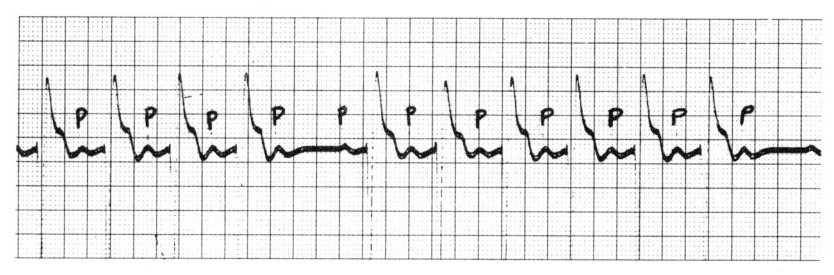

Figure 3-52. Mobitz Type II. Second degree heart block 7:6.

    Rate: Atrial 100; ventricular 86
    Rhythm: Regular — irregular
    P waves: Present; every seventh P wave is not followed by a QRS complex
    P-R interval: 0.35 second (prolonged)
    QRS complex: Normal

Arrhythmia present: Second degree heart block with a 7:6 block (7 P waves for every 6 QRS complexes)

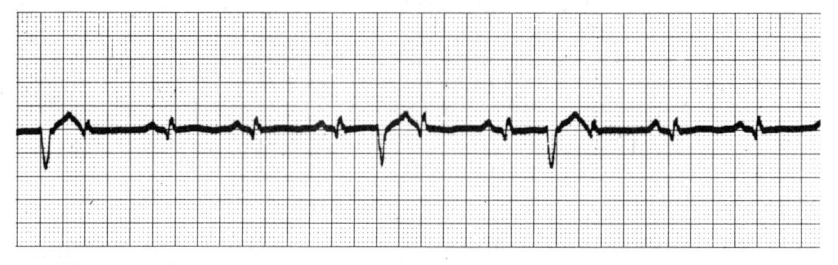

Figure 3-53. Normal sinus rhythm with interpolated PVCs.

Rate: 80-90
Rhythm: Irregular
P waves: Present; some P waves are absent before QRS complexes
P-R interval: 0.18 seconds (normal)
QRS complex: Normal, except for the first, sixth, and ninth complexes
Arrhythmia present: Normal sinus rhythm with interpolated PVCs
The premature ventricular contraction falls between two normal beats and is not followed by a compensatory pause
Note: The normal beats that follow each PVC are partially obscured by them.

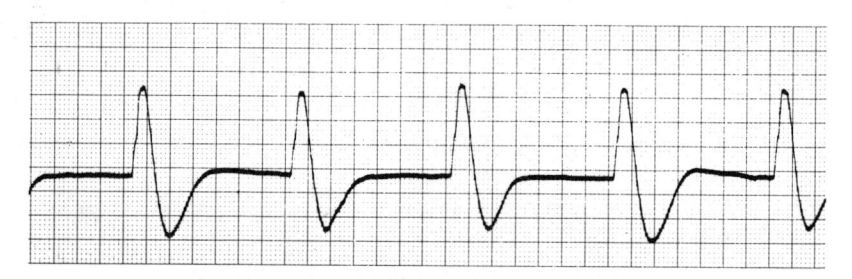

Figure 3-54. Idioventricular rhythm.

ARRHYTHMIAS

Rate: 46
Rhythm: Regular
P waves: Absent
P-R interval: Unidentifiable
QRS complex: Widened and slurred
Arrhythmia present: This slow ventricular rhythm is called an idioventricular rhythm

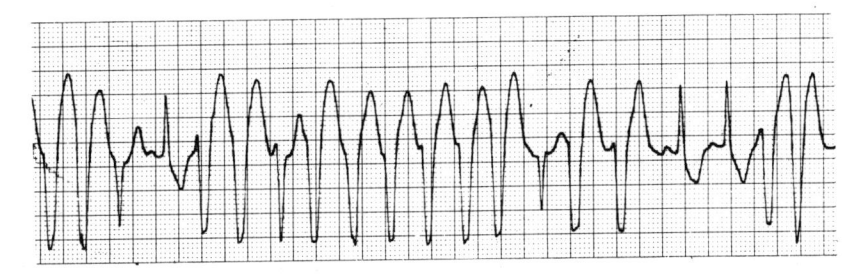

Figure 3-55. Ventricular tachycardia with normally conducted sinus beats.

Rate: Approximately 188
Rhythm: Irregular
P waves: Only the fourth, seventeenth, and eighteenth beats are preceded by P waves
P-R interval: 0.14 seconds (normal when P waves are present)
QRS complex: Widened and slurred except for the fourth, seventeenth, and eighteenth beats
Arrhythmia present: Ventricular tachycardia with occasional normally conducted sinus beats

CHAPTER 4

Pacemakers

DEFINITION AND HISTORICAL DEVELOPMENT

Artificial cardiac pacing is the maintenance of an adequate heart rate by direct electrical stimulation of the myocardium. Historically, as early as the nineteenth century attempts were made to stimulate the heart by the direct application of electrical current. However, there was not much progress in this area of cardiology until early in the twentieth century. In 1925 closed chest cardiac pacing was first accomplished by placing electrodes on the outside of the chest to provide electrical stimulation to the heart. The first use of a pacing electrode sutured to the myocardium was in 1957. It was inserted during cardiac surgery and attached to an external pacemaker. In 1959, cardiac pacing was successfully accomplished by implanting a transvenous electrode into the right ventricle by way of the venous system; by 1960, a completely implantable pacemaker had been developed.

USES

When the sinoatrial node is no longer able to pace the heart adequately, a pacemaker may be used to treat the severe bradycardia that would otherwise result in low cardiac output. Pacemakers are also used to slow very rapid atrial heart rates such as paroxysmal atrial tachycardia (PAT) and atrial flutter. These rapid rates are suppressed by the slower paced beats. Pacemakers are sometimes used in emergency situations to suppress certain ventricular arrhythmias. However, the *primary* purpose of cardiac pacing is to treat conduction defects that arise from a variety of causes—tissue necrosis, cardiac surgery, or congenital defects, for example.

TYPES OF PACEMAKER UNITS (PULSE GENERATORS)

External

The external pacemaker unit is a self-contained battery pack with output terminals to which the pacing electrodes are attached. On the face of the pacemaker are an output control for the milliampere setting, a rate control for the pulse setting, a visual indicator that signals each paced beat, and a sensitivity

PACEMAKERS

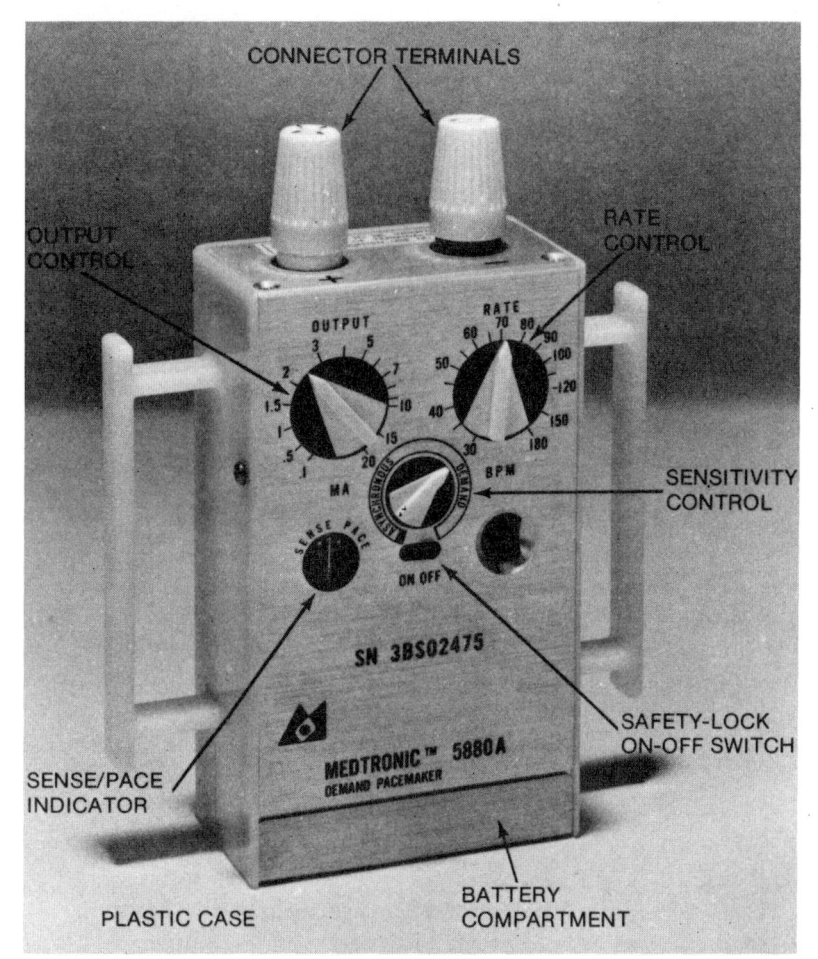

Figure 4-1. External demand pacemaker. Courtesy Medtronic, Inc.

control. The on and off switch is also located on the face of the pacemaker. This switch has a lock lever that must be manipulated with two hands, which prevents any accidental switching on or off of the pacemaker.

Internal

An internal pacemaker unit is used for permanent pacing. It is a small self-contained battery pack that is implanted internally in a surgically created subcutaneous pocket. It may be attached to either endocardial or epicardial electrodes for permanent pacing. Several models of permanent pacemakers are available, ranging from those that use mercury powered battery cells or lithium generated cells to those that use nuclear energy as their power source.

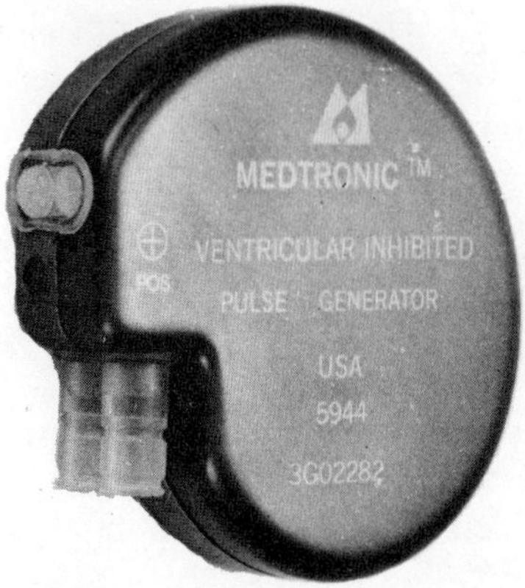

Figure 4-2. Internal pacemaker for permanent pacing. Courtesy Medtronic, Inc.

PACEMAKER RATES

Pacemaker rates are described as either "fixed" or "demand." The fixed-rate pacemaker provides an impulse at a set rate, usually between 60 and 80 beats per minute. It continues to pace at the preset rate until the batteries fail. This method of pacing is used infrequently, for while it provides the patient with a fixed, constant heartbeat it does not give the heart an opportunity to return to its own rhythm. Consequently, in patients who may have a temporary or intermittent conduction defect, any normally conducted heartbeats will be suppressed. In addition, competition between the artificial pacemaker and the patient's own heartbeat could occur if the pacemaker should malfunction and normal sinus rhythm has returned.

Demand pacemakers provide a more desirable method of pacing and are used more frequently. The pacemaker is set to fire when the patient's heart rate falls below a preset level. For example, if the pacemaker unit is set at 72 beats per minute, the pacemaker will begin to fire when the patient's own heart rate falls below 72. It will continue pacing without interruption until the patient's heart is again able to beat at least 72 times per minute. The demand pacemaker has the ability to sense ventricular contractions that result from normally conducted beats, and when they occur at a rate above that for which the pacemaker is set they prevent activation of the pacemaker. Conversely, the demand pacemaker will be automatically activated when the ventricles fail to contract.

Demand pacing is the most widely used pacing method because it allows the sinoatrial node to take over the pacemaking function whenever it is able to do so and allows for the greatest number of normally conducted beats possible. There is also less possibility of competition between the pacemaker and the patient's own heartbeat should restoration of the normal conduction activity of the heart occur.

Figure 4-3a is an example of the ECG in complete heart block, the most common arrhythmia for which pacemakers are used. The atrial rate is 75 beats per minute and the ventricular rate is irregular, between 50 and 80; three ventricular foci are firing. Figure 4-3b shows the change in the ECG following the insertion of a transvenous pacemaker. The atrial rate remains at 75 beats per minute, and the ventricles are being paced at a rate of 72 beats per minute.

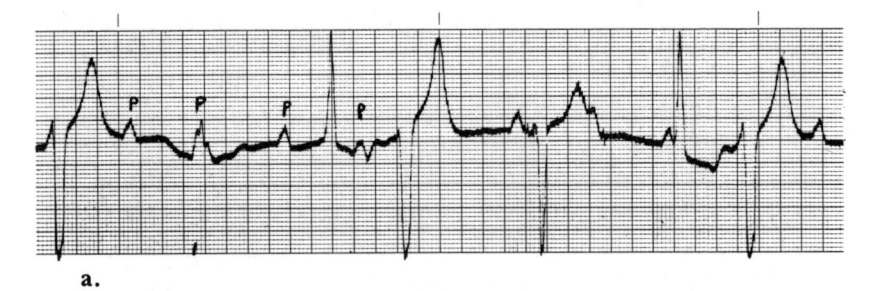

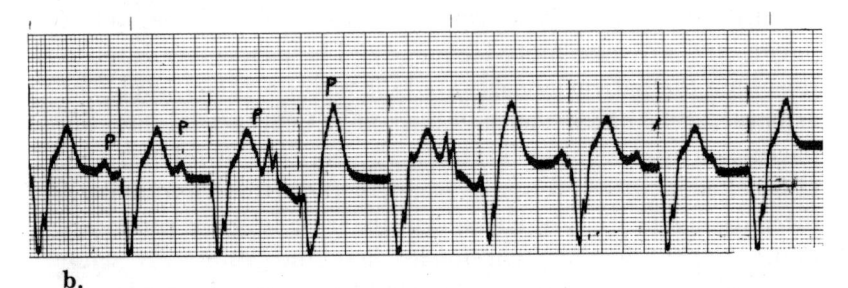

Figure 4-3, a and b. a. Example of the ECG in complete heart block. b. The ECG of the same patient as in (a) shows the change in the pattern following the insertion of a transvenous pacemaker.

PACEMAKER ELECTRODES

Epicardial Electrodes

Epicardial electrodes are usually used for permanent pacing. They are surgically implanted on the ventricular wall through a thoracotomy incision. The electrode wires are buried in the myocardial muscle and are usually attached to a pacemaker unit. An internal pacemaker is used when the electrodes have been implanted for permanent pacing. When epicardial electrodes are implanted at the time of cardiac surgery they may be attached to an external pacemaker until it is determined

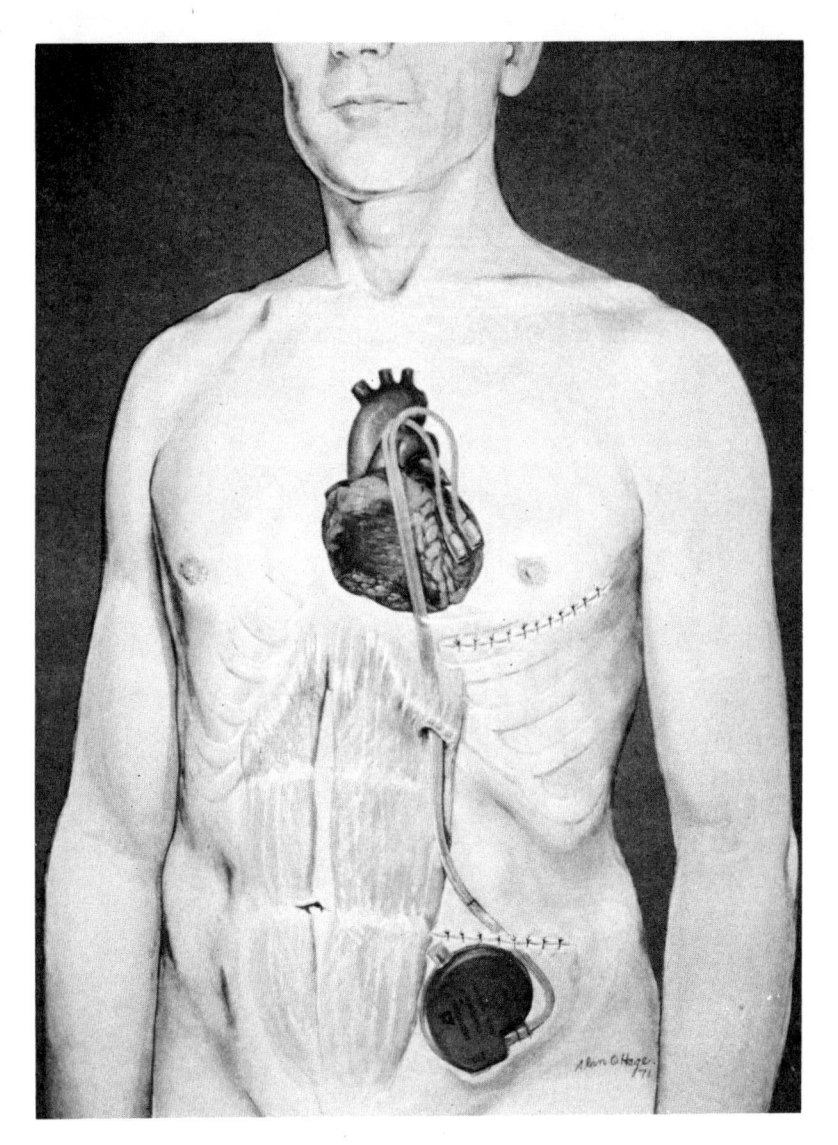

Figure 4-4. Internal pacemaker with surgically implanted epicardial electrodes. Courtesy Medtronic, Inc.

whether permanent pacing is needed. Epicardial electrodes are used infrequently because of the greater effectiveness of endocardial (transvenous) pacing.

Endocardial Electrodes

Endocardial electrodes are passed into the heart transvenously, i.e., through the venous system (Figure 4-5).

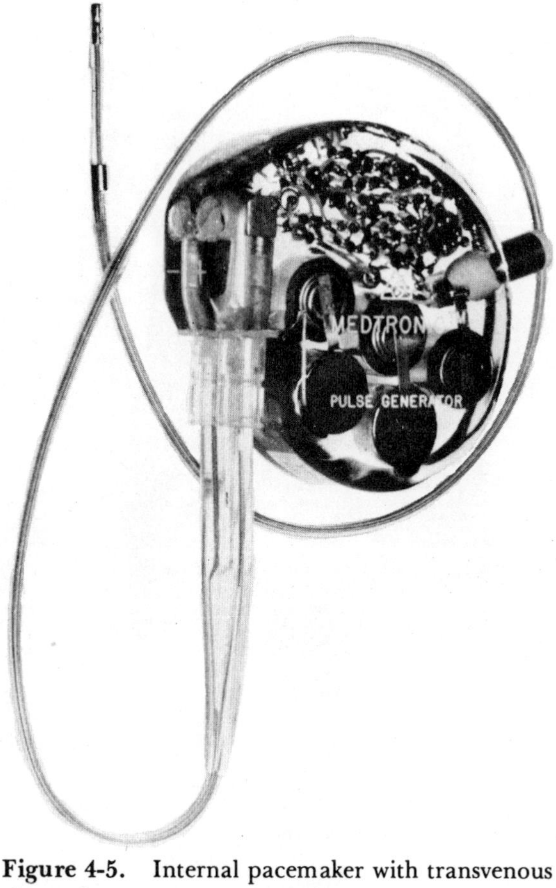

Figure 4-5. Internal pacemaker with transvenous (endocardial) electrode. Courtesy Medtronic, Inc.

PACEMAKERS

When temporary pacing is needed, the antecubital or the femoral vein is used (Figure 4-6).

When permanent pacing is needed, the electrode is inserted through the jugular or the subclavian vein (Figure 4-7).

For both temporary and permanent pacing, the passage of the electrode into the heart is done under fluoroscopy with the electrode being advanced until it reaches the apex of the right ventricle. In emergency situations, a semifloating endocardial electrode may be inserted, using electrocardiographic

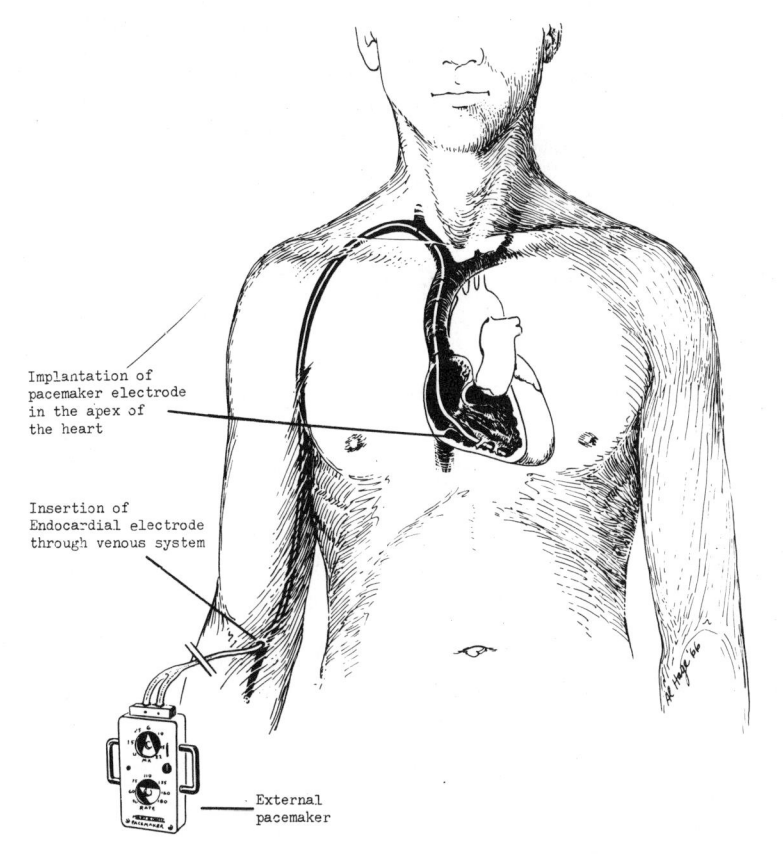

Figure 4-6. The electrode for a temporary pacemaker inserted through the antecubital vein. Courtesy Medtronic, Inc.

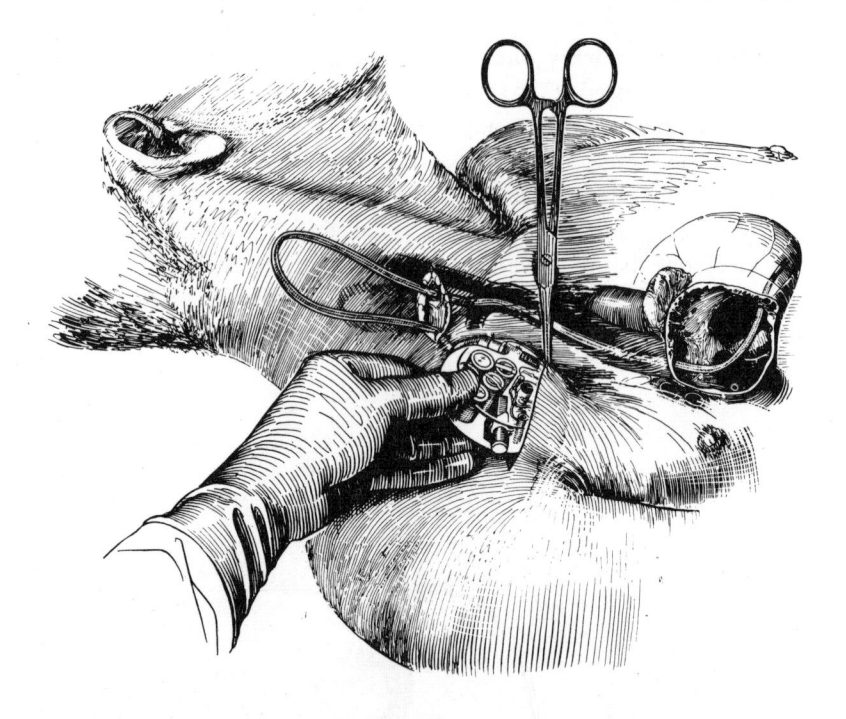

Figure-4-7. Method of implantation of a transvenous pacemaker. Courtesy Medtronic, Inc.

monitoring if fluoroscopy is not available. Changes in the ECG pattern are observed to determine when successful electrode placement is accomplished.

Transthoracic Electrodes

Transthoracic electrodes may also be used in emergency situations. In this instance, a large needle is passed either substernally or through the fourth or fifth intercostal space into the right or left ventricle. One end of a pacing electrode is passed through the needle into the ventricular cavity and the other end is attached to an external pacemaker. A transthoracic electrode is used when the emergency is such that a pacemaker is needed immediately. If the emergency is less critical and there is more than 15 minutes available for inserting the pacing catheter, an endocardial electrode will be used.

NURSING CARE OF PATIENTS WITH PACEMAKERS

The nursing care of patients with permanent pacemakers should begin prior to the insertion of the pacemaker. Since most patients will already have used a temporary pacemaker, they should be told why the permanent one is needed and how it will be inserted. A brief explanation of how the heart functions in response to electrical stimulation will provide the patient with a basis for further understanding. A description of the alteration that has occurred in the patient's regular electrical conduction system can lead to a discussion of how the pacemaker will help the heart to carry out its pumping function.

In general, the patient goes to the cardiac catheterization laboratory for implantation of a transvenous electrode that is connected to an external pacemaker unit. Teaching about the actual procedure should include a description of the room and the kinds of equipment the patient might see there—fluoroscopes and monitors, for example. The preanesthetic medication and local anesthetic that will be used should be discussed, as well as what will actually happen during the procedure. A description of the pacing electrode is also in order. Knowing the reasons for the presence of several doctors and nurses will help the patient to understand exactly what is going to happen to him. If an external pacemaker unit is available, the patient should be allowed to see and handle it.

Following insertion of the electrode, constant cardiac monitoring is needed to observe pacemaker function. When a fixed-rate pacemaker is used, a small artifact (often called the pacemaker blip or spike) should precede every QRS complex. This will indicate that every ventricular contraction has been stimulated by the pacemaker, and the pacemaker is said to be "in capture." The patient's pulse should not vary from the preset rate, and the number of QRS complexes should remain stable.

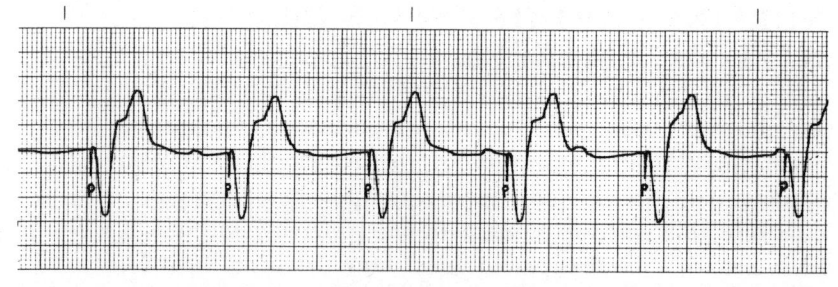

a.

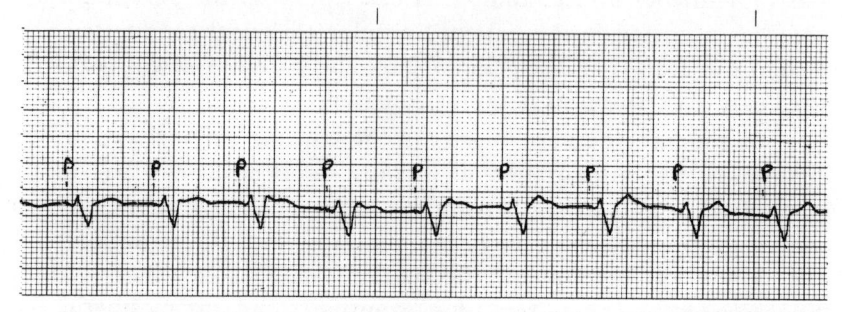

b.

Figure 4-8, a and b. Examples of the ECG when a pacemaker is in capture.

Occasionally, competition between the fixed-rate pacemaker and the patient's own heartbeat may occur. In this instance, the cardiac monitor will indicate that the pacemaker stimulus is competing with an occasional sinus beat or a premature ventricular contraction; this should be reported.

When a demand pacemaker has been inserted, the pacemaker artifact will not be present unless the patient's pulse falls below the rate at which the demand pacemaker has been set. For example, if the pacemaker has been set to pace when the patient's heart rate falls below 72, the ECG pattern will not show a pacemaker artifact unless the patient's own pulse falls below 72. When this occurs, the pacemaker will be activated and an artifact will be seen until the patient's own heart rate is 72 or above. It must be remembered that a patient who has a demand pacemaker will probably have an ECG pattern that is slightly irregular, since some beats are paced and some are unpaced.

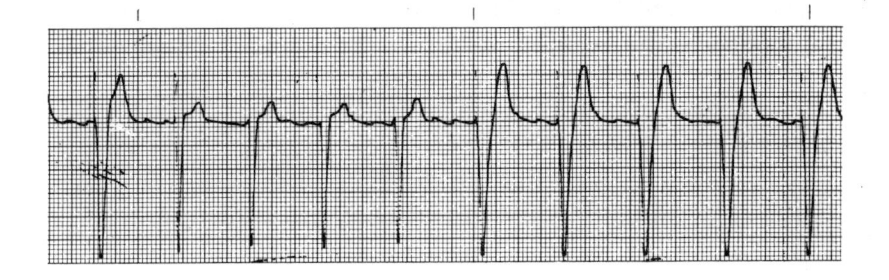

Figure 4-9. The ECG of a patient with a demand pacemaker that fires only when the heart rate falls below a preset level of 84.

During the first few days following the insertion of a pacemaker, the tip of the pacing catheter may become dislodged. When this occurs, the pacemaker will no longer be in capture. That is, a pacemaker artifact may be seen on the cardiac monitor; however, it will not be followed by a QRS complex. Clinically, the patient may begin to have the same signs and symptoms he had prior to the insertion of his pacemaker. Other disturbances in the cardiac rhythm may occur as a result of myocardial sensitivity to the pacing catheter. These

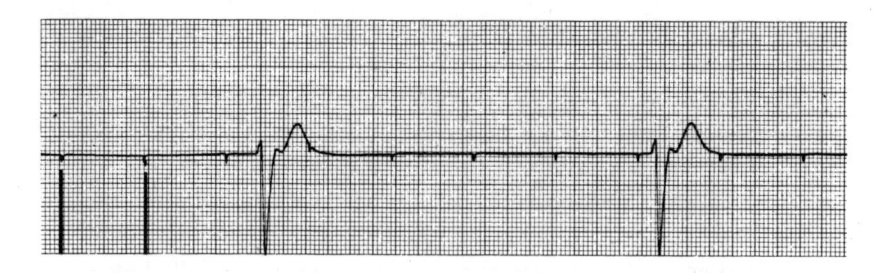

Figure 4-10. Example of the ECG when the pacemaker is out of capture. The pacemaker is firing but the pacemaker artifacts are not followed by ventricular beats.

include occasional PVCs or runs of ventricular tachycardia. Any of these changes in rhythm must be reported. In some hospitals the nurse is the one who will adjust the rate and voltage on the external pacemaker unit in the absence of the physician.

Another important function of the nurse in the patient care unit is the elimination of all electrical hazards. Under normal conditions, the tissue that surrounds the body provides a high degree of resistance to the passage of electrical current. When a person has an external transvenous pacemaker, the pacing electrode provides a low resistance pathway directly to the heart. In this situation, any stray current from ungrounded electrical equipment such as a lamp or radio, or from an improperly grounded plug, could follow this low resistance pathway to the heart and result in ventricular fibrillation. It is the nurse's responsibility to be sure that all equipment in the patient's room is properly grounded and that three-pronged adapters, often called "cheaters," have not been used. The reason for these precautions should be explained to the patient, especially if any personal articles such as a radio or a tape recorder must be removed from his room. In addition to these precautions, the exposed electrodes at the end of the pacing catheter should be insulated at the site of their insertion into the external pacemaker. A light-colored rubber glove may be used for this purpose, since it will protect the pacing wires from becoming wet and still provide visualization of the dials on the pacemaker unit.

Another problem that may arise in the patient who has an external pacemaker is phlebitis, or infection at the site of insertion of the pacing electrode. This may be prevented by the daily application of an antibiotic ointment and a small, dry sterile dressing to the site of insertion. The area may be cleansed with an antiseptic soap and water every day provided that the ends of the pacing electrode that are attached to the pacing unit are well protected.

Preventing the breakage or dislodgment of the pacing catheter is another important nursing function. The extremity into which the pacing electrode has been placed should be immobilized. The use of an armboard will prevent elbow movement while allowing the fingers to be freely mobile. Limited passive range of motion exercises may be given to the shoulder to prevent stiffness.

The nurse should be constantly aware that perforation of the right ventricular wall may occur following pacemaker implantation. Although this complication is not always easily detected, it should be considered when there is evidence that the pacemaker is no longer in capture or when there appears to be regular spasm of the lower chest or upper abdomen. Cardiac tamponade rarely occurs as a result of ventricular perforation; however, if such signs and symptoms of cardiac tamponade as low blood pressure, increased pulse, cyanosis, restlessness, and distended neck veins are seen, it is essential that the physician be notified immediately.

Occasionally, patients with a transient heart problem need a temporary pacemaker for only a short period of time. In such an instance, the patient must be given an adequate explanation of why the pacemaker is necessary and why it may eventually be removed. If psychological dependence on the pacemaker occurs, reassurance and support must be given to lessen the patient's anxiety when it is removed.

Most patients who require a temporary transvenous

pacemaker will need a permanent pacemaker. The preoperative teaching prior to permanent pacemaker insertion should include a description of what will happen on the day of surgery, teaching the patient to cough and deep breathe, and answering his questions about the procedure. In addition, several facts must be explained thoroughly, as the patient who is to have a permanent pacemaker will have it for the rest of his life and, indeed, the length of his life may depend on its proper functioning.

The way the heart functions and the patient's need for a pacemaker may have to be reviewed with him. Although this information was undoubtedly explained previously, the patient frequently denies the actual need for a permanent pacemaker hoping that the temporary unit will provide a cure. If possible, a used pacemaker or a model provided by a manufacturer should be shown to the patient. This will give him an opportunity to see the actual size of the pacemaker, to touch it, and to feel its weight. If the model is encased in clear plastic, the patient will be able to see the batteries and examine the working parts. The actual placement of the pacemaker should be explained preoperatively. For most women, the pacemaker will be inserted under the breast and will be well hidden when a slightly larger brassiere is worn. For male patients, the pacemaker is usually implanted in the area of the axilla. If the patient engages in a particular sport—hunting, for example—the physician should be informed in advance so that at the time of surgery the pacemaker can be placed in an area that will not be adversely affected by the use of a gun.

If epicardial electrodes are being used with implantation directly on the wall of the myocardium, preoperative preparation should be similar to that for any patient having a thoracotomy. The patient should be informed that the pacemaker battery pack will probably be implanted in the abdominal area.

During the postoperative period the same observations of the cardiac rhythm for pacemaker function are followed as after implantation of an external transvenous pacemaker (see page

82). The same types of postoperative problems may also occur, and any changes in the ECG or in the patient's condition should be reported to the physician. Care of the surgical wound is similar to that for any surgical wound, keeping in mind that the battery pack (pacemaker) is a foreign object implanted under the skin. The usual signs of infection should be watched for and proper reporting initiated. The patient's attitude about his pacemaker is important to consider. There is no need for the patient to fear the pacemaker since it will allow him to increase his activity rather than limit it. Since the patient with a pacemaker may tire a little more rapidly that he did before, the level of his activity may be limited. Nevertheless, he will be able to resume any activities appropriate to a person of his age and interests, such as golfing, swimming, or jogging. Contact sports must be avoided, however. Shoulder movement and active range of motion are encouraged following the insertion of the permanent pacemaker to prevent stiffness of the shoulder.

The electrical hazards associated with the use of an external pacemaker are not present because the battery pack for the permanent pacemaker is insulated under the skin. Once the wound is healed, the hazards associated with water are also eliminated and the patient may shower or take a tub bath. Electrical appliances may be used with the exception of microwave (radar range) ovens. Since these ovens adversely affect the proper functioning of the pacemakers, they must be avoided. Patients should be reminded that microwave ovens are frequently installed in cafeterias and canteens that have self-service machines. Others hazards include airport radar, some power lawnmowers, large power-plant generators, and high-voltage electrical fields. Some of the newer pacemaker models are no longer inhibited by some of this equipment, so the type and model of pacemaker should be investigated before giving this information to patients. Airport screening devices will not adversely affect the pacemaker; however, the pacemaker may set off an alarm system.

Pacemaker failure is inevitable because the life of the

batteries is limited to 24 to 36 months, depending on the model of pacemaker being used. Teaching the patient to take his pulse for a full minute daily, and to report any significant changes in rate, has been one of the suggested methods of checking for pacemaker failure. The patient should understand that if his pulse falls below the preset level, his physician should be notified. For example, if a patient has a pacemaker set at 72 beats per minute and his pulse falls to 66, he should call his doctor immediately since he will need to have his pacemaker examined and possibly replaced. Some cardiologists no longer consider this method of detecting pacemaker malfunction the best one for determining pacemaker failure. Many now recommend that the patient be examined every 2 to 3 months and the pacemaker evaluated by placing a magnet over the battery pack. The magnet is designed to convert a demand pacemaker to a fixed-rate pacemaker, which will allow evaluation of the state of the batteries. Most patients can check their own pacemaker every day by using an inexpensive transistor radio. When the radio is set at 550 kc, turned on, and placed over the pacemaker, it will produce a click before every heartbeat initiated by the pacemaker. If this method is used, an increase or decrease of five beats per minute in the pulse rate, or any noted irregular beats should be reported to the physician. In some geographic areas, pacemaker function can be checked by the use of a telephone monitor. In this instance, the pacemaker artifact and the patient's peripheral pulse are transmitted by telephone using a bipolar probe and a plethysmograph. This allows evaluation of the functioning of the pacemaker at a testing facility so that patients who live long distances from a medical center can have accurate evaluation of their pacemakers.

Other important points in patient teaching prior to discharge include:

1. Reminding the patient to report any return of the symptoms he had prior to receiving his pacemaker.

2. Telling the patient that travel is not restricted but that he should inform his physician before he leaves and request a list of physicians or hospitals he might contact in an emergency.
3. Providing him with a pacemaker identification card or information about Medic-Alert.
4. Explaining to the patient that sexual activity may be resumed. Female patients contemplating pregnancy may be told that their pacemaker will not interfere with pregnancy or harm the child in any way.
5. Telling the patient that all physicians or dentists he may consult must be told about the pacemaker before any treatment is initiated. The use of diathermy or any other device which uses an electrical current may adversely affect the pacemaker.

The development and improvement of pacemakers in the last several years has been very rapid and their use has become commonplace. Future advances will certainly take place, and the nurse who cares for patients with cardiac pacemakers must be alert to innovations and their effect on nursing practice.

SELF TEST

The following section contains both questions for review and rhythm strips for self-testing. The answers to these exercises may be found at the end of the section.

QUESTIONS FOR REVIEW

1. What is the difference between sinus tachycardia and sinus bradycardia?
2. How do sinus tachycardia and sinus bradycardia differ from normal sinus rhythm?
3. What is the difference between sinus tachycardia and paroxysmal atrial tachycardia?
4. What is absent on the ECG when sinus arrest occurs?
5. Where does the pacemaker wander in wandering pacemaker?
6. What is the cause of sinus arrhythmia? Is it a serious arrhythmia?
7. Compare atrial fibrillation and atrial flutter.
8. What happens to the P wave in junctional (nodal) rhythms?
9. What is the only ECG change when first degree heart block is present?
10. Describe the ECG change that occurs in second degree heart block.
11. What does a diagnosis of "second degree 4:1 block" mean?
12. Describe what happens in complete heart block.
13. What are the major characteristics of a PVC?
14. What occurs in ventricular tachycardia?
15. What happens to the P waves when a patient is in ventricular tachycardia?
16. Describe the ECG in ventricular fibrillation.

RHYTHM STRIPS FOR SELF-TESTING

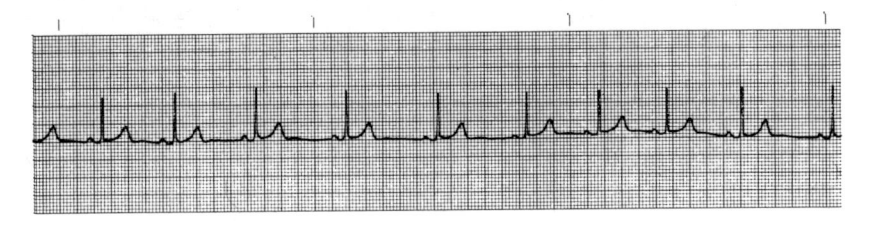

Rhythm Strip 1

Rate:
Rhythm:
P waves:
P-R interval:
QRS complex:
Arrhythmia present:

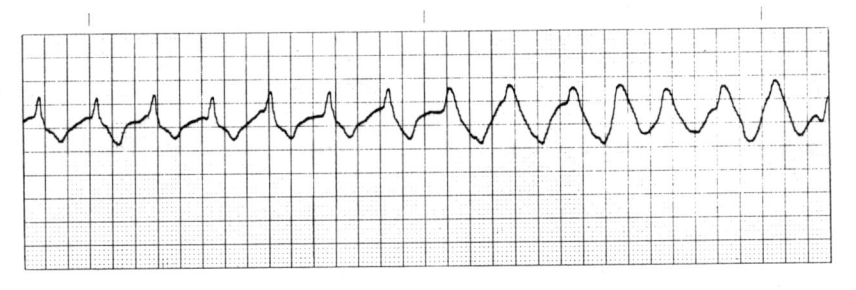

Rhythm Strip 2

Rate:
Rhythm:
P waves:
P-R interval:
QRS complex:
Arrhythmia present:

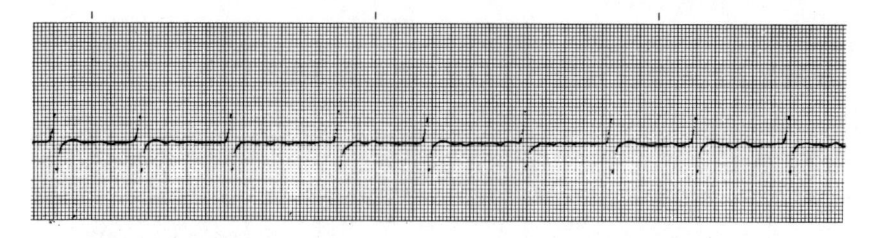

Rhythm Strip 3

Rate:
Rhythm:
P waves:
P-R interval:
QRS complex:
Arrhythmia present:

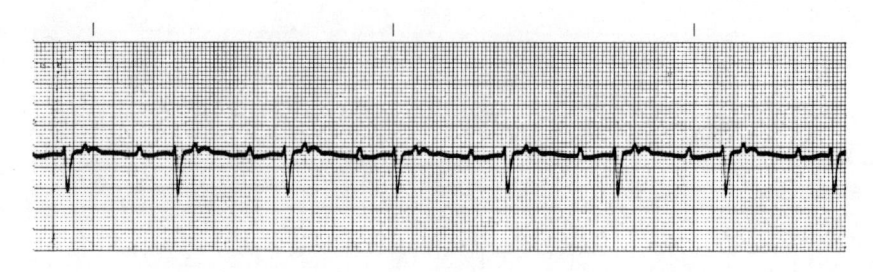

Rhythm Strip 4

Rate:
Rhythm:
P waves:
P-R interval:
QRS complex:
Arrhythmia present:

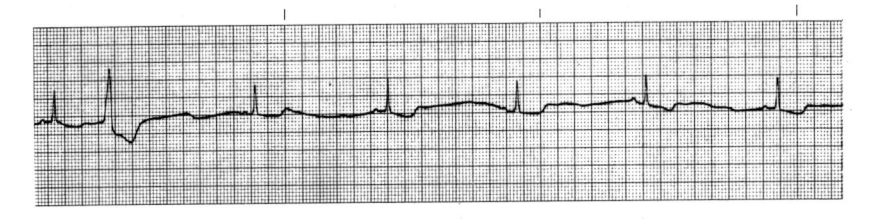

SELF TEST 95

Rhythm Strip 5

Rate:
Rhythm:
P waves:
P-R interval:
QRS complex:
Arrhythmia present:

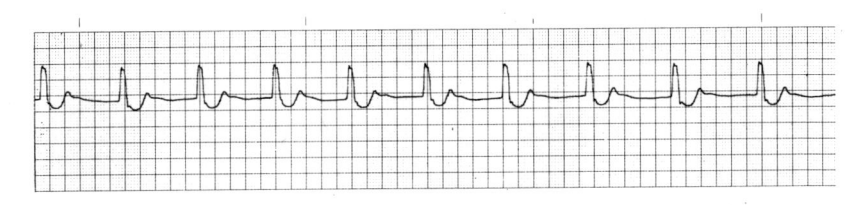

Rhythm Strip 6

Rate:
Rhythm:
P waves:
P-R interval:
QRS complex:
Arrhythmia present:

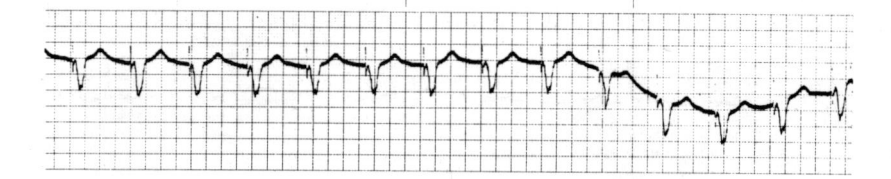

Rhythm Strip 7

Rate:
Rhythm:
P waves:
P-R interval:
QRS complex:
Arrhythmia present:

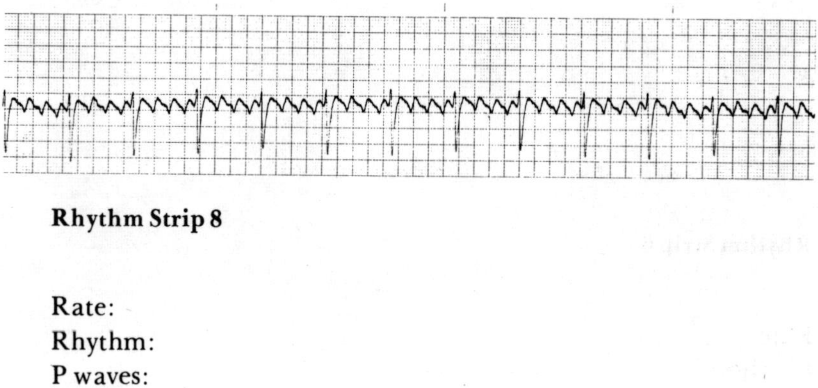

Rhythm Strip 8

Rate:
Rhythm:
P waves:
P-R interval:
QRS complex:
Arrhythmia present:

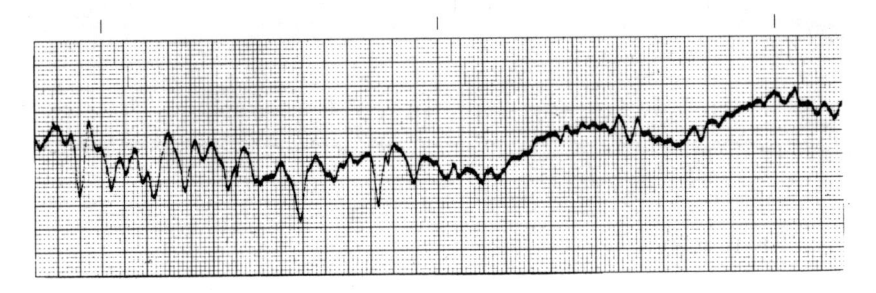

SELF TEST

Rhythm Strip 9

Rate:
Rhythm:
P waves:
P-R interval:
QRS complex:
Arrhythmia present:

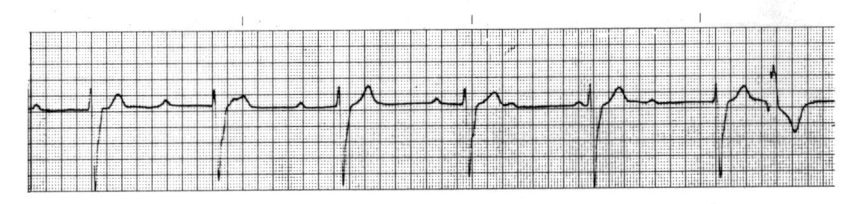

Rhythm Strip 10

Rate:
Rhythm:
P waves:
P-R intervals:
QRS complex:
Arrhythmia present:

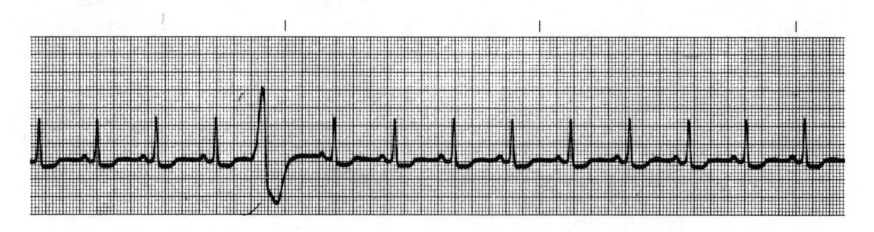

Rhythm Strip 11

Rate:
Rhythm:
P waves:
P-R interval:
QRS complex:
Arrhythmia present:

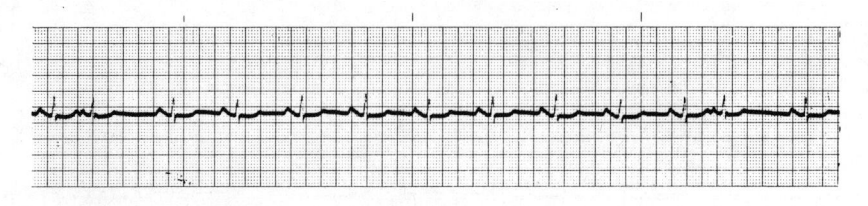

Rhythm Strip 12

Rate:
Rhythm:
P waves:
P-R interval:
QRS complex:
Arrhythmia present:

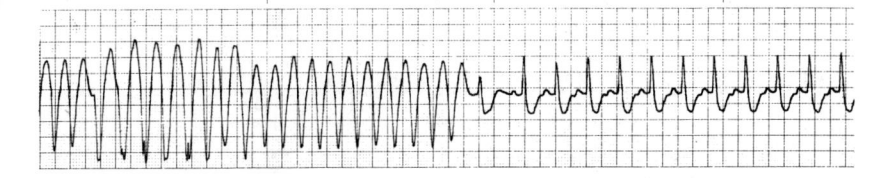

SELF TEST

Rhythm Strip 13

Rate:
Rhythm:
P waves:
P-R interval:
QRS complex:
Arrhythmia present:

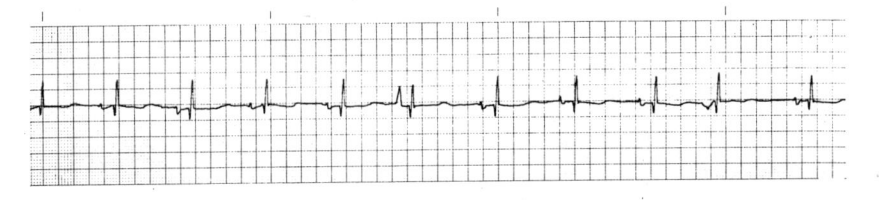

Rhythm Strip 14

Rate:
Rhythm:
P waves:
P-R interval:
QRS complex:
Arrhythmia present:

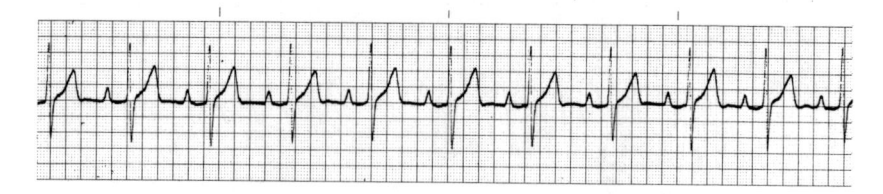

Rhythm Strip 15

Rate:
Rhythm:
P waves:
P-R interval:
QRS complex:
Arrhythmia present:

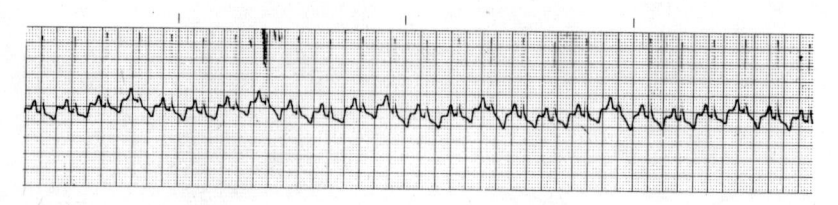

Rhythm Strip 16

Rate:
Rhythm:
P waves:
P-R interval:
QRS complex:
Arrhythmia present:

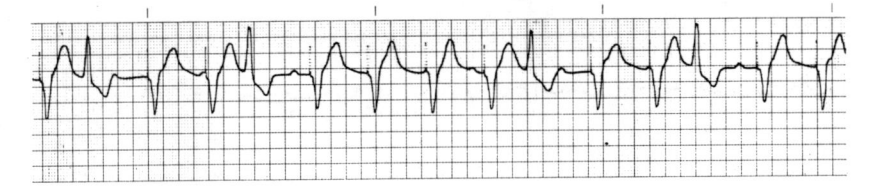

SELF TEST

Rhythm Strip 17

Rate:
Rhythm:
P waves:
P-R interval:
QRS complex:
Arrhythmia present:

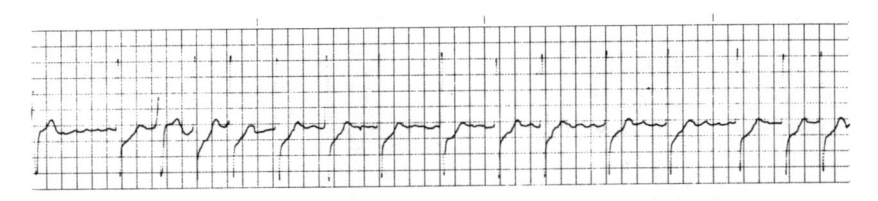

Rhythm Strip 18

Rate:
Rhythm:
P waves:
P-R interval:
QRS complex:
Arrhythmia present:

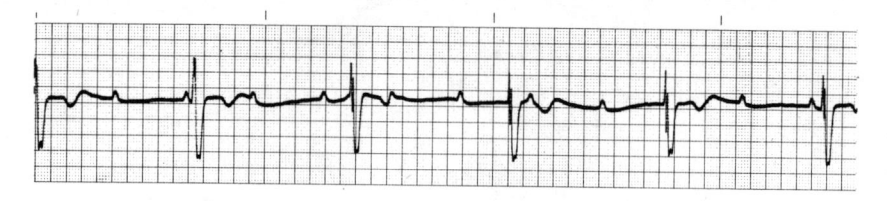

SELF TEST

Rhythm Strip 19

Rate:
Rhythm:
P waves:
P-R interval:
QRS complex:
Arrhythmia present:

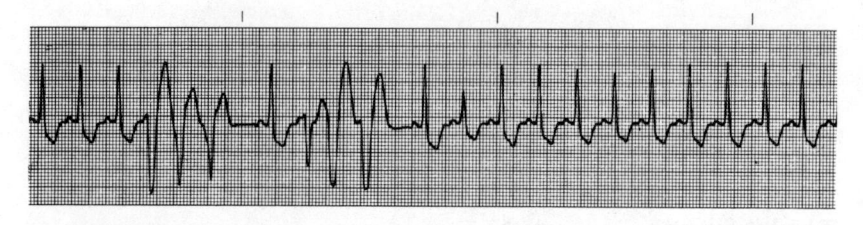

Rhythm Strip 20

Rate:
Rhythm:
P waves:
P-R interval:
QRS complex:
Arrhythmia present:

Answers to Review Questions

1. The only difference between sinus tachycardia and sinus bradycardia is the rate. Sinus tachycardia is characterized by a rapid sinus rhythm and sinus bradycardia by a slow sinus rhythm.
2. Sinus tachycardia and sinus bradycardia differ from normal sinus rhythm in rate alone. Sinus tachycardia is usually defined as a rate of over 100 beats per minute (between 100 and 180) and sinus bradycardia is usually defined as a rate below 60 beats per minute.
3. Sinus tachycardia originates in the sinoatrial node at a rate between 100 and 180 beats per minute, while paroxysmal atrial tachycardia (PAT) originates from an ectopic focus in one of the atria at a rate between 160 and 250 beats per minute.
4. In sinus arrest a complete complex (the P, Q, R, S, and T waves) is absent.
5. In wandering pacemaker, the pacemaker wanders from the sinoatrial node throughout the atria to the atrioventricular junction (node).
6. Sinus arrhythmia is most commonly associated with respirations. There is an increase in heart rate on inspiration and a decrease on expiration. This is a normal physiological variant and usually is of no clinical significance.
7. In atrial fibrillation there are several ectopic foci or circus movements attempting to take over the pacing function of the heart; this results in a grossly irregular ventricular rate with an absence of P waves and the presence of fibrillation waves.

    In atrial flutter there is one ectopic focus or circus movement attempting to take over the pacing function of the heart. The ventricular rate is variable and may be regular, regularly irregular, or grossly irregular depending on the degree of block present. P waves are absent and saw-toothed flutter waves are seen on the ECG.

8. In junctional (nodal) rhythms the P waves are either inverted before or after the QRS complex or buried within it.

9. When first degree heart block is present the only abnormality on the ECG is a prolonged P-R interval.

10. In second degree A-V block some but not all of the impulses are conducted by the A-V junction (node). The P-R interval may be normal or prolonged.

11. In a second degree 4:1 A-V block only one out of every four beats is conducted to the ventricles through the A-V junction (node).

12. In complete heart block the atria and ventricles beat independently of each other with no beats being conducted through the A-V junction (node).

13. The major characteristics of a PVC are:
    The beat occurs prematurely
    The beat is followed by a full compensatory pause
    The QRS complex is widened and slurred
    There is no P wave preceding the QRS complex
    The T wave is in the opposite direction from the QRS complex.

14. In ventricular tachycardia an ectopic focus in the ventricles paces the heart faster than 100 beats per minute.

15. In ventricular tachycardia P waves are present because the S-A node is still attempting to pace the heart; however, they are usually buried in the QRS complex and are not easily identifiable.

16. In ventricular fibrillation the ECG pattern shows a completely erratic, bizzare rhythm in which there are no identifiable P, Q, R, S, or T waves.

Identification of Rhythms

Rhythm Strip 1
    Rate: 60–75
    Rhythm: Irregular
    P waves: Normal
    P-R interval: 0.16 seconds (normal)
    QRS complex: Normal
    Arrhythmia present: Sinus arrhythmia

Rhythm Strip 2
    Rate: 150
    Rhythm: Regular
    P waves: Absent
    P-R interval: Unidentifiable
    QRS complex: Widened and slurred
    Arrhythmia present: Ventricular tachycardia

Rhythm Strip 3
    Rate: 53–68
    Rhythm: Irregular
    P waves: Absent; fibrillation waves present
    P-R interval: Unidentifiable
    QRS complex: Normal
    Arrhythmia present: Atrial fibrillation

Rhythm Strip 4
    Rate: Atrial 107; ventricular 55
    Rhythm: Regular
    P waves: Present; every other P wave is not followed by a QRS complex
    P-R interval: 0.36 seconds (prolonged)
    QRS complex: Normal
    Arrhythmia present: Second degree 2:1 A-V block

Rhythm Strip 5
>Rate: 40
>Rhythm: Basic rhythm is regular except for first, second, and third complexes
>P waves: Present except for second complex
>P-R interval: 0.12 seconds (normal)
>QRS complex: Normal except for second complex which is widened and slurred, premature, and followed by a compensatory pause (this pause is not a *full* compensatory pause)
>Arrhythmia present: Sinus bradycardia with one premature ventricular contraction (PVC)

Rhythm Strip 6
>Rate: 60 (slight increase toward end of strip)
>Rhythm: Regular
>P waves: Buried in QRS complex: seen as notch on "R" wave
>P-R interval: Unidentifiable
>QRS complex: Normal
>Arrhythmia present: Midjunctional (nodal) rhythm

Rhythm Strip 7
>Rate: 80
>Rhythm: Regular
>P waves: Absent; straight line (artifact) precedes every QRS complex
>P-R interval: None
>QRS complex: Widened and slurred
>Arrhythmia present: A paced rhythm. Pacemaker stimulus (artifact) seen before every QRS complex

SELF TEST

Rhythm Strip 8
    Rate: Atrial 300; ventricular 75
    Rhythm: Regular
    P waves: Saw-toothed flutter waves
    P-R interval: Unidentifiable
    QRS complex: Normal
    Arrhythmia present: Atrial flutter with a 4:1 block

Rhythm Strip 9
    Rate: Indeterminable
    Rhythm: Indeterminable
    P waves: Absent
    P-R interval: None
    QRS complex: None; irregular wave-like oscillations present
    Arrhythmia present: Ventricular fibrillation

Rhythm Strip 10
    Rate: Atrial 62; ventricular 36
    Rhythm: Regular
    P waves: Present but unrelated to QRS complexes
    P-R interval: Absent
    QRS complex: Widened and slurred, last complex originating from a different focus than others on strip
    Arrhythmia present: Complete (third degree) heart block with two ventricular foci

Rhythm Strip 11
>Rate: 88
>Rhythm: Basic rhythm is regular
>P waves: Present, except before fifth complex
>P-R interval: 0.16 seconds (normal)
>QRS complex: Normal except for fifth complex which is widened and slurred, premature, and followed by a full compensatory pause
>Arrhythmia present: Normal sinus rhythm with one premature ventricular contraction (PVC)

Rhythm Strip 12
>Rate: 75
>Rhythm: Basic rhythm is regular except for second and twelfth complexes which are premature and followed by compensatory pauses
>P waves: Present
>P-R interval: 0.20 seconds (normal)
>QRS complex: Normal
>Arrhythmia present: Normal sinus rhythm with two premature atrial contractions (PACs)

Rhythm Strip 13
>Rate: Incalculable on first half of strip; 150 on second half
>Rhythm: Indeterminable on first half of strip; regular on second half
>P waves: Absent on first half of strip; present on second half
>P-R interval: None on first half of strip; 0.16 seconds (normal) on second half
>QRS complex: Wave-like oscillations on first half of strip; normal on second half
>Arrhythmia present: Ventricular flutter with spontaneous conversion to sinus tachycardia

SELF TEST

Rhythm Strip 14
    Rate: 60
    Rhythm: Regular (occasionally a slight variance of 0.12 seconds)
    P waves: Present; shape varies; some are inverted
    P-R interval: 0.20 seconds with occasional variance depending on origin of P wave
    QRS complex: Normal
    Arrhythmia present: Wandering atrial pacemaker

Rhythm Strip 15
    Rate: 58-60
    Rhythm: Regular
    P waves: Normal
    P-R interval: 0.28 seconds (prolonged)
    QRS complex: Normal
    Arrhythmia present: First degree A-V block, rate falls slightly below 60 (sinus bradycardia) in some places

Rhythm Strip 16
    Rate: 150
    Rhythm: Regular
    P waves: Present
    P-R interval: 0.12 seconds (normal)
    QRS complex: Normal
    Arrhythmia present: Sinus tachycardia

Rhythm Strip 17
    Rate: 78
    Rhythm: Irregular
    P waves: None present; artifact present before most QRS complexes
    P-R interval: Unidentifiable
    QRS complex: Widened and slurred; occasionally upright and normally shaped
    Arrhythmia present: Demand pacemaker with occasional normal sinus beats

Rhythm Strip 18
    Rate: Between 70 and 80
    Rhythm: Irregular
    P waves: None present; fibrillation waves seen
    P-R interval: Unidentifiable
    QRS complex: Normal
    Arrhythmia present: Atrial fibrillation

Rhythm Strip 19
    Rate: Atrial 65, ventricular 30
    Rhythm: Regular
    P waves: Present, but unrelated to QRS complexes
    P-R interval: Unidentifiable
    QRS complex: Widened
    Arrhythmia present: Complete (third degree) A-V block

SELF TEST

Rhythm Strip 20
    Rate: 136
    Rhythm: Regular at beginning and end of strip; irregular in middle of strip
    P waves: Present before first, third, seventh, and last eleven QRS complexes
    P-R interval: 0.12 seconds (normal) when P waves are present
    QRS complex: Normal except for fourth, fifth, and sixth, and eighth, ninth, and tenth complexes
    Arrhythmia present: Sinus tachycardia with short bursts of ventricular tachycardia (three PVCs in a row)

SELECTED READINGS

Books

Andreoli, K.G., Fowkes, V.H., Zipes, D.P. and Wallace, A.G.
    Comprehensive Cardiac Care, 3rd ed., St. Louis, C.V. Mosby, 1975
Bellett, S. *Essentials of Cardiac Arrhythmias,* Philadelphia: Saunders, 1972
Chung, E.K. *Electrocardiography,* Hagerstown Md., Harper and Row, 1974
Conway, N. *A Pocket Atlas of Arrhythmias.* London, Wolfe Medical, 1974
Fontaine, G., Grosgogeat, Y. and Welti, J.J. *The Essentials of Cardiac Pacing,* London, Heinemann Medical, 1976
Fowler, N.O. *Cardiac Arrhythmias.* Hagerstown Md., Harper and Row, 1977
Ganong, W.F. *Review of Medical Physiology,* 8th ed., Los Altos, Ca., Lange Medical Publications, 1977
Goldman, M.J. *Principles of Clinical Electrocardiography,* 9th ed., Los Altos, Ca., Lange Medical Publications, 1976
Guyton, A. *Textbook of Medical Physiology,* 4th ed., Philadelphia, Saunders, 1971
Habner, P. *Nurses' Guide to Cardiac Monitoring,* 2nd ed., London, Balliere Tindall, 1975
Hamer, J. *An Introduction to Electrocardiography,* Tunbridge Wells, Pitman Medical, 1975
Julian, D.G. and Oliver, M.F. *Acute Myocardial Infarction,* Edinburgh, Churchill Livingstone, 1968
Kernicki, J., Bullock, R. and Matthews, J. *Cardiovascular Nursing,* New York, Putnam, 1970
Netter, F.J. *Heart—the Ciba Collection of Medical Illustrations,* Summit, N.J., Ciba Publications, 1969

SELECTED READINGS

Meltzer, L.E. and Dunning, A.J. *Textbook of Coronary Care*, Amsterdam, Excerpta Medica, 1972

Meltzer, L.E., Pinneo, R. and Kitchell, J.R. *Intensive Coronary Care*, 3rd ed., Bowie Md., Charles Press, 1977

Pantridge, J.F., Adgey, A.A.J., Geddes, J.S. and Webb, S.W. *The Acute Coronary Attack*, Tunbridge Wells, Pitman Medical, 1975

Sanderson, R.G. *The Cardiac Patient*, Philadelphia, Saunders, 1972

Schamroth, L. *An Introduction to Electrocardiology*, 5th ed., Oxford, Blackwell Scientific Publications, 1976

Stock, J.P.P. and Williams, D.O. *Diagnosis and Treatment of Cardiac Arrhythmias*, 3rd ed., London, Butterworths, 1974

Journal Articles

Adgey, A.A.J., Allen, J.D., Geddes, J.S., James, R.G.G., Webb, S.W., Zaidi, S.A. and Pantridge, J.F. 'Acute Phase of Myocardial Infarction,' *Lancet*, ii, 501-4, Sept., 1971

Bigger, J.T., Dresdale, R.J., Heissenbuttel, R.M., Weld, F.M. and Wit, A.L. 'Ventricular Arrythmias in Ischaemic Heart Disease. Mechanism, Prevalence, Significance and Management', *Progress in Cardiovascular Diseases*, 19, 255-300, Jan./Feb., 1977

Coulshed, N. '*Heart Block*', Part 1, *Nursing Times*, 74, 149-53, Jan., 1978

Coulshed, N. '*Heart Block*', Part 2, *Nursing Times*, 74, 190-93, Feb., 1978

Hoffman, F. and Cranefield, P. 'The Physiological Basis of Cardiac Arrhythmias', *American Journal of Medicine*, 37, 670-84, 1964

Julian, D.G., Valentine, P.A. and Miller, G.G. 'Disturbances of Rate Rhythm and Conduction in Acute Myocardial Infarction,' *American Journal of Medicine*, 37, 915-26, 1964

Krikler, D.M. 'A Fresh Look at Cardiac Arrhythmias', Part I, *Lancet*, i, 851-4, 1974

Krikler, D.M. 'A Fresh Look at Cardiac Arrhythmias', Part II, *Lancet*, i, 913-8, 1974

Krikler, D.M. 'A Fresh Look at Cardiac Arrhythmias', Part III, *Lancet*, i, 974-6, 1974

Krikler, D.M. 'A Fresh Look at Cardiac Arrhythmias', Part IV, *Lancet*, i, 1034-1937, 1974

Lown, B., Vassaux, C., Hood, W.B., Fakhro, A.M., Kaplinsky, E. and Roberge, G. 'Unsolved Problems in Coronary Care', *American Journal of Cardiology*, **20**, 494-508, 1967

Mogensen, L. 'Ventricular Tachyarrhythmias and Lignocaine Prophylaxis in Acute Myocardial Infarction', *Acta Medica Scandinavica*, Suppl. 513, 1-80, 1970

GLOSSARY

action potential the electric current that is set up in a muscle or other excitable tissue during its activity; the combination of depolarization and repolarization of the cell membrane

aorta the main trunk of the arterial system; it arises in the left ventricle and carries oxygenated blood away from the heart to the rest of the body

arrhythmia an abnormality in the rate, rhythm, or conduction of the heartbeat

artery a vessel that carries blood away from the heart to the various parts of the body; with the exception of the pulmonary artery, arteries carry oxygenated blood

arteriole a small artery

artifact any wave or mark on the electrocardiographic tracing that does not represent part of the cardiac cycle; it is caused by the technique used and is merely incidental

atrium one of the two upper chambers of the heart

atrial refers to an atrium

atrioventricular bundle (bundle of His) part of the conduction system of the heart; consists of a bundle of neuromuscular tissue that originates in the atrioventricular node, passes through the atrioventricular junction and downward along the interventricular septum, and finally divides into the right and left bundle branches that are distributed to the right and left ventricles

atrioventricular (A-V) dissociation describes the condition that exists when the atria and ventricles beat independently of each other; each beats in response to its own pacemaker

atrioventricular node a small node of specialized tissue located on the lower right part of the interatrial septum; transmits the impulse that arises in the S-A node to the ventricles, delaying it slightly so that the atria have a chance to empty before the ventricles contract

atrioventricular valves the valves located between the atria and ventricles on both the right and left sides of the heart; they control the flow of blood through the atria and ventricles

bicuspid valve *see* mitral valve

block the slowing or stoppage of an impulse when it is traveling toward a given point

bundle of His *see* atrioventricular bundle

capillary a microscopic vessel that connects an arteriole and a venule

circus movement term applied to a continuous movement of an excitation wave that arises in an ectopic focus and travels in a circular fashion around a ring of muscle within the atrial wall so that only part of the impulse is conducted to the ventricle

chordae tendinae fibrous cords that join the cusps of the atrioventricular valves to the papillary muscles

conduction system consists of the S-A node, A-V junction (node), bundle of His, right and left bundle branches, and the Purkinje fibers; it is the system that conducts the impulses throughout the heart to produce the heartbeat

coronary arteries the arteries (right and left) that supply blood to the heart itself

depolarization stimulation of a resting cell resulting in a change in the polarity of the cell membrane

ectopic beat a heartbeat that arises from a pacemaker in the heart other than the S-A node

electrocardiogram (ECG) a graphic recording of the changes in the electrical potential that occur during the heartbeat

GLOSSARY

endocardium the membrane that lines the chambers of the heart and covers the cusps of the various heart valves

epicardium the inner layer of the pericardial sac that is in contact with the heart

His's bundle *see* atrioventricular bundle

inferior vena cava the great vein that carries venous blood from the lower part of the body to the right atrium

mitral valve the two-cusped valve located between the left atrium and the left ventricle; it allows blood to flow freely from the atrium into the ventricle and prevents backflow from the ventricle into the atrium during ventricular contraction

myocardium the muscular substance of the heart

nonrefractory period the period in the cardiac cycle during which cells are polarized and able to accept stimuli

P wave the electrocardiographic wave that represents depolarization of the atria

P-R interval the period of time from the beginning of atrial depolarization to the beginning of ventricular depolarization as recorded electrocardiographically

pacemaker *see* sinoatrial node

papillary muscles extensions of the muscular wall of the ventricles that give rise to the chordae tendinae

pericardium the double-layered fibroserous sac that encloses the heart

premature beat heartbeat arising from an ectopic focus before the beat that results from the normal stimulus from the S-A node

pulmonary artery the artery that carries unoxygenated venous blood from the right ventricle to the lungs

pulmonary veins the veins that carry oxygenated blood from the lungs to the right atrium

Purkinje fibers the terminal fibers of the right and left bundle branches; they form a network that extends into the subendocardial tissue of both ventricles, carrying electrical stimuli from the atria to the ventricles

QRS complex the electrocardiographic pattern that represents depolarization of the ventricles

refractory period the period during which cells are depolarized and unable to accept a stimulus

repolarization reestablishment of the resting potential of a cell membrane following depolarization

retrograde conduction movement of impulses through the conduction system in a direction that is the reverse of the normal conduction pattern

septum a wall or partition; the atrioventricular septum is a muscular wall that divides the heart into the right and left sides; the interatrial septum separates the two atria; the interventricular septum separates the two ventricles

sinoatrial node (S-A node) the pacemaker of the heart; consists of a collection of specialized tissue in the wall of the right atrium where the contraction of the heart is initiated

superior vena cava the great vein that carries venous blood from the upper part of the body to the right atrium

supraventricular impulse an impulse that arises in any portion of the heart above the ventricles (S-A node, atria, A-V junction, or above the point of bifurcation of the bundle of His)

tricuspid valve the three-cusped valve located between the right atrium and right ventricle; it allows blood to flow freely from the right atrium into the right ventricle and prevents backflow of blood from the ventricle into the atrium during ventricular contraction

T wave the electrocardiographic wave that represents ventricular depolarization during which time the ventricles are in a relative refractory period

vein a blood vessel through which blood is returned to the heart; with the exception of the pulmonary veins, veins carry dark or unoxygenated blood

GLOSSARY

ventricle one of the two thick, muscular lower chambers of the heart that pump blood out of the heart

venule a small vein